# YOU DON'T LOOK SICK

## QUICK AND DIRTY TIPS FOR SURVIVING ULCERATIVE COLITIS

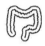

## A.W. CROSS

GLORY BOX PRESS

You Don't Look Sick: Quick and Dirty Tips for Surviving Ulcerative Colitis

Cover illustration by Peter Cross
Cover design by germancreative
Book design and production by Glory Box Press
Editing by Mia Darien

A.W. Cross
gloryboxpress@gmail.com

Printed in Canada

First Printing: May 2016

ISBN 978-1-7751787-2-9

Although the author and publisher have made every effort to ensure that the information in this book was correct at press time, the author and publisher do not assume and hereby disclaim any liability to any party for any loss, damage, or disruption caused by errors or omissions, whether such errors or omissions result from negligence, accident, or any other cause.

This book is not intended as a substitute for the medical advice of physicians. The reader should regularly consult a physician in matters relating to his/her health and particularly with respect to any symptoms that may require diagnosis or medical attention.

# ABOUT THE AUTHOR

A.W. Cross is a Canadian writer and blogger. She has experienced the entire gamut of what ulcerative colitis has to offer, from diagnosis to j-pouch. Whenever she has time, she enjoys her family, friends, and anything even remotely to do with food.

You can follow her on Facebook @thescreamingmeemie or visit her website, screamingmeemie.com

*You Don't Look Sick: Quick and Dirty Tips for Surviving Ulcerative Colitis* is her first book.

**Other Titles in the *Quick and Dirty Tips for Surviving* Series:**

*My Other Bag's a Prada: Quick and Dirty Tips for Surviving an Ileostomy*
*Unicorn Farts and Glitter: Quick and Dirty Tips for Surviving a J-Pouch*

For all of you who live with ulcerative colitis: you're nails.

# CONTENTS

# PREFACE

I was diagnosed with ulcerative colitis in 2009 after a long, nearly fatal process of testing and trials. The next few years of my life were like falling through the Looking Glass as I fumbled my way through the haze of near-constant flares. I became privy to a new way of life, and I discovered previously untapped resources in myself and others: endurance, empathy, and the ability to bend so, so far without breaking.

Being able to find the humor, however black, in my condition was perhaps the greatest revelation of all. In a culture that is so impatient with chronic illness, being able to laugh at the very thing that gave me so much grief allowed me to keep what few shreds of sanity and dignity I had left.

So in 2015 (now sans colon), I joined the NaNoWriMo rebellion, and I wrote what would eventually become three books—this is the first. Writing about what I've learned during my illness also inspired me to found my IBD blog, screamingmeemie.com

I hope this book makes you laugh, and I hope you find it practical. Most of all, I hope it helps you realize that even though your illness may be invisible at times, you most definitely are not.

AW Cross, 2016

# INTRODUCTION

"It's just a stomach bug." These are often the words spoken by the naïve individual just before their unstoppable descent into the bloody, excrement-filled abyss that is ulcerative colitis.

Some among us will be affected so acutely that their colons will be sliced from their bodies in a haze of morphine and lime Jell-O®, leaving them free at last from endemic attack but scarred and forever condemned to a life of inhibited flatulence. They are the lucky ones. The less fortunate will linger for years in the paralyzing clutches of the Flare, a cyclical nightmare of pain, diarrhea, and hope, with no savior but the double-edged sword of The Corticosteroid, upon which they must impale themselves without mercy.

There is no cure; even those who have had their organs excised and resectioned will bear the consequences throughout their lives. Is this affliction then an obstacle that cannot be overcome? An end to a worthy quality of life? Shall we simply give up and succumb to its insidious cruelty?

No.

Although it cannot be conquered in full, ulcerative colitis can be subdued, brought to heel, and assimilated. It can be survived, and survived with style.

That is why this book was written: to help prepare you for making ulcerative colitis your bitch. This book is not for the self-pitying, or for the determined invalid. It is for those whose illness will not define them, who laugh in the face of the colonoscope, and who realize that, even in a diaper, they're still sexy as hell.

The symptoms, diagnosis, and treatment of ulcerative colitis are not covered here—there are sufficient other resources for that. This book is about what comes after that initial attack. This is your battle plan. From this book, you will learn the basic maneuvers of coping with the physical and emotional aspects of ulcerative colitis, the intermediate theory of fashion choices, survival kits, and hospital etiquette, and the more advanced tactics of dealing with other people's ignorance and using social media to discuss your illness.

All of the knowledge provided here has been hard-won by personal experience. Know that struggling is not failing, and in this war, there is no definitive victory; it will last a lifetime. The wisdom provided in this book may not always lead you to triumph, but it will give you an arsenal to draw from. The rest is up to you.

See you on the other side.

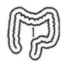

# ULCERATIVE COLITIS

## YOU DON'T LOOK SICK

### THE DARK CLOUD

Unless you are an inhumanly positive person, you've probably noticed that ulcerative colitis has some downsides, especially during a flare. The physical anarchy—to say nothing of the emotional mayhem—can fool you into thinking that ulcerative colitis is The Big Bad. Some of its more dastardly ploys include:

**FLARES**
Near-constant diarrhea, gut-clenching abdominal pain, and alabaster-brow-inducing blood loss.

**THE NEED FOR CORTICOSTEROIDS**
Crazy pills that make you more erratic than the cat lady down the street. Angry? Happy? Sad? Hungry? Confused? Tired? Giddy? It must be Wednesday.

**FATIGUE**
Your days have 32 hours now.

**GOODBYE BUTT SKIN**
No, you didn't accidentally wipe yourself with steel wool, but your skin's peeled off just the same.

### DEHYDRATION
For every pint of water you drink, three will come out.

# THE SILVER LINING

But, just like the antagonist in any great story, even ulcerative colitis has its good side:

### GOODBYE CONSTIPATION
Well, for most of us. Inexplicably, sometimes people with ulcerative colitis still get constipated, especially when they are in remission. In general, though, you'll never have to strain again!

### GET OUT OF JAIL FREE
Okay, not literally. But now you have this awful chronic illness. You feel dreadful, and you need to make sure that everyone around you knows it. For maximum impact, put less emphasis on the diarrhea aspect and more on the internal bleeding (which can sound incredibly romantic in a Victorian sort of way). Smile bravely. The next time your friend requests you attend her product party, all you have to do is assume a look of wistful regret and gracefully decline. You have a good excuse not to go, and she can't say a thing against you without looking like a stone-cold bitch. WARNING: Use sparingly, or people will stop inviting you to events you actually want to go to.

### LEGAL, MEDICAL-GRADE DRUGS
You can now take the trip you were always too scared/uptight/broke to take. If you have to take them anyway, you may as well relax and enjoy it. Responsibly.

### SPECIAL BATHROOM ACCESS
Get the key, get the card, get the app, whatever. And use it. Waiting in line is for suckers.

### COMFORTABLE ABSENCE OF SELF-CONSCIOUSNESS
Always wanted to stroll in all your naked glory through the changing room at the pool but were too shy? The sheer indignity of your

symptoms and the procedures involved in treating your ulcerative colitis will gift you a whole new yardstick with which to measure bodily shame. This perk may take time to develop, but it's incredibly liberating when it does finally happen.

## SMUGNESS
In the knowledge that you are hard-as-nails. Ulcerative colitis is a constant battle. You know how to *endure*.

## BUTT PLAY
If interested, you now have the opportunity to engage in an act that you may have considered previously illicit with no self-censure: the opportunity to have an attractive man/woman (GIs tend to be a good-looking lot) stick their fingers into your behind. If you're into that sort of thing, you've won the lottery. If you're not, then life's about to get awkward.

## SYMPATHY SWAG
People love to buy sympathy gifts when someone they love is ill. Always be grateful and don't abuse people's kindness by asking for things like a car. Accept graciously. That sixth copy of the Kama Pootra is just as special as the first.

## YOU'VE JOINED AN EXCLUSIVE CLUB
Having ulcerative colitis automatically grants you membership into a special community full of potential allies. Granted, there may be better commonalities with which to bind people together, but there are also worse. Just look at the Putney High Tide Club.

## LITERACY
You'll finally learn how to spell diarrhea. Probably.

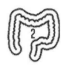

# I CAN'T FEEL MY FACE

## PHYSICAL CONSEQUENCES OF ULCERATIVE COLITIS AND HOW TO COPE

### PHYSICAL CONSEQUENCES OF ULCERATIVE COLITIS

You've discovered by now that there are a lot of physical consequences associated with ulcerative colitis, and none of them are pleasant:

**DIARRHEA**
When you're in remission, you'll probably go only as often as you did before you became ill. During a flare, you may have up to forty (sometimes more) bowel movements a day.

**NAUSEA**
The colitis itself can make you nauseous, and nausea is also a common side effect of your medication.

**FATIGUE**
You will be tired from the illness itself and as another side effect of your treatment.

**PAIN**
Abdominal pain, headaches, joint pain, perianal pain… If it can hurt,

chances are, it will.

## WEIGHT FLUCTUATIONS

Between fearing to put anything in your mouth during a flare to wanting to put everything in your mouth when you are in remission, you will likely find your weight goes up and down. Steroid therapy can also give you extra heft.

## ANEMIA

In ulcerative colitis, anemia is usually due to iron deficiency through blood loss.

## DEHYDRATION

Water is absorbed via the colon, and the more inflamed your colon, the less water you'll be able to absorb.

## MALNUTRITION

Although the majority of nutrients are absorbed in your small bowel, you may not much feel like eating. Plus, those foods that are usually the easiest for you to eat often don't have the highest nutritional value.

## MOUTH SORES

Both the illness and steroid therapy can cause persistent mouth ulcers.

## HEMORRHOIDS AND FISSURES

Frequent bowel movements can result in hemorrhoids and splits in your anal skin. You'll literally get a crack in your crack.

## OTHER VARIOUS SIDE EFFECTS OF YOUR MEDICATION

The side effects can often make you feel worse than the ulcerative colitis itself and may include symptoms such as insomnia, night terrors, confusion, and the overwhelming desire to punch someone in the face.

## INFLAMMATION OF OTHER ORGANS

Ulcerative colitis can cause inflammation in your skin, eyes, joints, and bile ducts.

## ARTHROPATHIES

You may find you develop an arthritis, such as ankylosing spondylitis, in the long term.

## BONE LOSS

Bone loss is caused by steroid treatment and can become quite severe if not treated.

# POTENTIAL COMPLICATIONS

If you are especially unlucky, you might experience complications that can become serious or even life-threatening without medical attention. Complications of ulcerative colitis can include:

## FISTULAS

Although rare in ulcerative colitis, if the inflammation in your colon is particularly severe, you may develop a fistula (an opening between two organs).

## PERFORATED COLON

The inflammation in your colon may become so severe it creates a hole in your intestinal wall.

## SEVERE BLOOD LOSS

You can pass so much blood during a flare that you may require a blood transfusion.

## INFECTION

The inflamed patches and abscesses present when your disease is active can be vulnerable to bacterial infections such as *C.difficile*.

## TOXIC MEGACOLON

A potentially life-threatening condition that can result in colon perforation and sepsis.

## COLON CANCER

Ulcerative colitis doesn't give you colon cancer, but it does increase your risk of developing it.

# TIPS FOR COPING

All of these consequences can be difficult to cope with, especially if you were in robust health before you developed ulcerative colitis. People deal with their symptoms in different ways, whether for good or for bad, but there do seem to be common successful strategies. It is obviously more difficult to cope in the midst of a flare than it is when you are in remission, and since you feel so much better when you are in remission, it's tempting to let any preemptive strategies slide. Don't. One of the best ways of coping during a flare is to be proactive when you are in remission—you may not be able to prevent a flare, but you can help lessen the severity and improve your ability to survive it successfully. It's boring as hell, but it does work. If nothing else, a proactive strategy will help you to avoid the inevitable self-blaming and emotional flagellation of "if only I had done more" that can occur with a flare.

## DURING REMISSION

When you are in remission, ensure that you keep yourself as healthy as possible:

### EAT A REASONABLY HEALTHY DIET

Although what you eat will not prevent a flare, a decent diet will help your body cope better when it does happen.

### EXERCISE

I know, BORING. But just do *something*, even if it's only walking to the pub. Like diet, exercise will not prevent flares, but it will improve your ability to cope with them.

## TAKE THE TIME TO DE-STRESS

Stress is thought to play a role in triggering flares as it prompts your immune system to get all uppity, so make time to do nothing. This may be easier said than done, especially if you're the kind of person who finds doing nothing stressful. The key is to think of it as something important and necessary. If you make relaxing part of your regular routine, you will eventually find it easier to switch off.

## GET ENOUGH SLEEP

This one may be easier to accomplish, thanks to the fatigue. A lack of sleep results in stress, and you know how that ends.

## ALWAYS TAKE YOUR SURVIVAL KIT WITH YOU

Or, at the very least, make sure it's close at hand. Peace of mind = less stress = clinging to remission just a little bit longer.

## TAKE YOUR MEDICATION AS PRESCRIBED

Don't be that person who thinks that they're the one being who magically doesn't have to take their medication, who then gets a severe flare and has the bloody cheek to moan about it. Nobody likes that person.

## BE AWARE OF ANY TRIGGERS

If you can, avoid particularly stressful situations that may contribute to triggering a flare. Unfortunately, sometimes your body will react to any strong emotion, including happiness, as though it were stress. Try not to have feelings of any kind.

## TAKE YOUR MULTI-VITAMINS

Stock up on anything that may be depleted by a flare or your medication, such as potassium and calcium.

# DURING A FLARE

No matter what you do to prevent it, you will eventually have another flare. Take the following steps to ensure you survive it:

## KNOW THE WARNING SIGNS
Since the warning signs are subtle in the initial stages, identifying them early may take you a couple of flares. Eventually, though, you'll develop a sixth sense about it. Pay attention and act accordingly.

## DON'T WAIT TO INFORM YOUR DOCTOR
Even if you have a supply of medication at hand, let your doctor know your ulcerative colitis is active so they can keep a record. It is also useful to keep a flare diary yourself. Keeping track of how often your flares occur and their duration will indicate any need for changes in, and the future implications for, your treatment.

## KNOW WHEN TO GO TO HOSPITAL
There are no gold stars for bravery in ulcerative colitis; a perforated colon is the only reward you'll get if you wait too long to seek treatment. If your pain is particularly severe, or you have a fever, get your inflamed ass to the hospital.

## BATHROOM RECONNAISSANCE
When you are out and about, make sure you know where the bathrooms are located, so if you need to make a mad dash, you can at least know you're going in the right direction. Apps for your phone, such as Bathroom Finder, will map out the location of the bathrooms in your current venue. Unfortunately, the area has to have been previously surveyed to be of any use. Also, don't wait until the last second to download/use it.

## TELL YOUR BOSS
You'll likely be needing some time off work, and it's best to be upfront about your condition. Some bosses will be sympathetic, some will not.

## PIMP OUT YOUR BATHROOM
You're going to be spending a lot of time in there, so you may as well make it pleasant.

## KEEP SURVIVAL KITS EVERYWHERE

If you have several squirreled away, you won't have to worry about forgetting it. Keep one at work, one in the car, one in your purse. Confidence!

## REST

Getting more rest should be obvious, but you may feel obligated to continue as normal. Accept that you can't. Pushing yourself often makes you feel worse and your flare last longer. Sometimes you just have to say 'f—- it' and relax. Saying it out loud helps a lot.

## GET LOTS OF SLEEP

Sleeping in the bathtub can be helpful if your flare is particularly bad. Load up your tub with pillows and blankets, and rest easy. Sometimes the knowledge that you don't have to go crashing down the hall at 3:00 am is enough to make you relax and sleep better.

## TAKE ANTIDIARRHEALS

Use only as prescribed, however, and never take them if you are bleeding. Bulking agents often work just as well, providing a soft mass to your stool that will naturally slow things down without stopping them.

## AVOID SIGNIFICANT FIBER

Take a hiatus from raw vegetables and other high-fiber foods as these will exacerbate your symptoms. You won't be digesting them anyway, and nothing will scare you in the middle of the night as badly as the sight of undigested bean sprouts in the toilet bowl.

## EAT

It's tempting not to eat during a flare—less in, less out—but you can become malnourished easily, and you'll lack the stamina to cope effectively with your flare. Eat small and often. Many people find that bland, softer foods help. Think low residue. If you're really struggling, buy some meal replacement drinks. They're nasty, but they'll help keep you nourished.

## APPLY HEAT

Put a hot pad (within the manufacturer's guidelines, of course) on your abdomen to help with the cramps. A soak in the tub is also good, just don't stay in too long. Your perianal skin is probably pretty delicate at this point and doesn't need the extra moisture.

## WEAR LOOSE, SOFT CLOTHING

Pajamas, yoga pants, whatever. Anything with a gentle elastic waistband. Dresses are good too, but lack the same snuggle factor.

## WIPES

Use baby wipes instead of toilet paper, and dab, don't wipe. Once you are clean, gently pat yourself dry with either gauze or a soft (purpose-designated) towel.

## POOP IN THE SHOWER

You'll reach a point during a flare when you are passing only liquid and blood, and even the breeze of dropping your pants is excruciating to your battered skin. When this happens, going to the bathroom in the shower can be a sanity saver. It takes minutes to clean the shower, days to rebuild your skin. Pat yourself dry between bouts. Anyone who judges you has clearly never been that ill and therefore is not allowed an opinion.

## VASELINE®, DIAPER RASH CREAM, WHATEVER

Use cream. Barrier creams are great as long as they work, but you need to re-apply them if they've been wiped off. Tedious, but worth it. Your skin will break down much faster than it will heal.

## DEVELOP A FLARE ROUTINE

Have a favorite book or movie? Best pair of pajamas? Put together a box of your favorite things to use during your flares. You may be surprised at how comforting the ritual is.

## GET A FLARE HOBBY, OR TWO

Cross-stitch, knit, play computer games. Your flare hobby should be something that you can do in bed or on the couch.

## PLAY THE SYMPATHY CARD

Don't forget to let everyone who loves you know how you're feeling, in a non-whiny way, of course. Sit back and wait for sympathy-swag and pity-love. **Warning:** Use in moderation.

# CAN'T WAIT: ACCESS TO PUBLIC BATHROOMS

Although knowledge about ulcerative colitis is increasing, the public services that support sufferers vary between countries.

Through Crohn's and Colitis UK, IBD patients in the United Kingdom are eligible for a *Can't Wait Card*: a wallet-size card which indicates the holder has a medical condition resulting in an urgency to use the bathroom. The cards encourage businesses to grant the holder access to washrooms that may not be available to the general public. Also available for UK patients is the *RADAR* key. Produced by the National Key Scheme, the key can be used to unlock public bathrooms all over the UK.

Crohn's and Colitis Australia also supports a *Can't Wait* program, which supplies cards to patients and *Can't Wait* stickers to businesses and retailers who display the stickers in their windows, indicating to cardholders that their toilets are available when needed.

*Can't Wait* cards are also available in the United States through the Crohn's and Colitis Foundation of America. At the time of writing, Canada's *Can't Wait* program is still in its infancy. Services currently available include the *GoHere Washroom Finder App*, which uses GPS to locate nearby washrooms and map out locations along a route of travel. While there is currently no physical *Can't Wait Card* in Canada, a virtual *GoHere Washroom Access Card* is available via the *Washroom Finder* app. A *GoHere* decal, similar to Australia's *Can't Wait* sticker, is being used on a trial basis in several Canadian cities, with plans to go nationwide if the pilot is successful.

# COPING WITH A FISTULA

Fistulas are not a common feature of ulcerative colitis, but they can occur if the inflammation in your bowel is severe enough. A fistula is essentially a tunnel that opens between your internal organs, or from an organ to the outside of your body. Types of fistulas that may occur with ulcerative colitis include:

- anal/perianal
- bowel to bladder
- bowel to vagina
- bowel to skin
- intestinal

Depending on your situation, your fistula may be treated with medications such as antibiotics, immunosuppressants, or biologics. Alternatively, it can be treated surgically with either a fistulotomy, fistulectomy, a seton stitch, or a LIFT procedure (ligation of the intersphincteric fistula tract). If these treatments fail, your doctor may recommend a permanent ostomy.

## TIPS FOR COPING WITH A FISTULA

### KEEP IT CLEAN

Keep the area around your fistula as clean and dry as possible. Wash around it using only warm water and disposable cloths or cotton wool to avoid introducing bacteria. When drying the skin around your fistula, dab, don't rub, to avoid irritating your skin. If you use a hairdryer to dry it, make sure you use the lowest setting.

### BATHE IT

If your fistula is uncomfortable, you may find a warm bath helps soothe it.

### DON'T PISS IT OFF

The chemicals in perfumed shower gels, soaps, powders, or lotions can irritate your fistula. Avoid using them around the area.

## BABY IT

To help avoid skin damage and irritation, apply a barrier cream wherever the drainage from your fistula comes into contact with your skin.

## LET IT BREATHE

Avoid wearing tight clothes and synthetic underwear. Think loose, soft cotton. Good air circulation will help to keep your fistula site dry.

## LET IT RELAX

You may find sitting painful at times. Take some pressure off your fistula by lying down. Avoid activities like bike-riding if you find it irritates your fistula.

## CUSHION IT

If you need to sit, sit on something soft. You can use a regular pillow or a purpose-made cushion. Sometimes even a thick sanitary pad is adequate.

## ABSORB IT

You may find you have leakage from your fistula. If so, use gauze, an incontinence pad, sanitary pad, or a pantyliner to help absorb the fluid.

## GIVE IT TIME

Fistulas can take months or even years to heal, which can be extremely disheartening and frustrating. Keep your expectations realistic.

## TALK ABOUT IT

Having a fistula is yet another kick in your already battered proverbial nuts. If you are struggling, get support, whether from a friend, a family member, or someone in your medical team.

## PREPARE FOR THE WORST

A fistula gives you an excuse to have yet another survival kit. Yay!

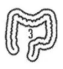

# BE PREPARED FOR HELL

## PLAN AHEAD

## ULCERATIVE COLITIS SURVIVAL KIT

Take inspiration from the Girl Guides/Scouts. One of the best ways to cope with your ulcerative colitis is to be prepared. A survival kit will give you peace of mind and can make the difference between an accident being a disaster or merely an inconvenience. It may seem excessive, but having a survival kit will give you the confidence to go out whenever and wherever you want, even during a flare.

### WIPES
Believe me, no matter how extra-soft/triple-ply/has-sewn-in-velvet-pillows that toilet paper is, it gets rough fast. Your skin can become so delicate during a flare that even the softest toilet paper will begin to feel like sandpaper. The best way to avoid this agony is with fragrance-free baby wipes for sensitive skin. And for your own well-being, dab, don't wipe. Don't forget to pat yourself dry afterward. It's not like you need extra moisture down there.

### VASELINE®
Vaseline®, or any other hypoallergenic petroleum-based lotion, acts as an excellent barrier between your poor, abused skin and all that liquid waste. Diaper rash cream also works well. After you're clean and dry, apply a modest amount.

**Bonus Tip:** Vaseline® makes extra-small tubs for lips, so a vat of it won't create a lot of bulk in your survival kit. Buy two if you're also going to be using it on your mouth.

## MENTHOLATED LOTION

After repeated effluvia-related insults, your perianal skin may become incredibly itchy. You definitely shouldn't scratch it, so your only options in this situation are to either wedge a pack of frozen peas between your cheeks or use a mentholated cream, such as Calmoseptine® or Gold Bond®. The menthol keeps everything nice and cool and, when used in combination with Vaseline®, the cream also acts as a barrier against further waste exposure. It's a win-win! Don't want to be minty-fresh? Any zinc-based diaper-rash cream will also help.

## ANTIDIARRHEALS

Immodium® (loperamide), or other antidiarrheals, can be extremely helpful in a pinch, especially if you happen to be on a road trip or in some other circumstance where you won't be able to dash to the toilet. Obviously, you'll have to plan to take your dose in advance, since it won't start working immediately.

## PAINKILLERS

For pain, obviously. Avoid ibuprofen, since it can further annoy your already irritated system.

## A CHANGE OF CLOTHES

It doesn't have to be a full change: it can just be clean underwear. Even if you have a near miss, you'll feel better if you can freshen up.

## JUST CHANGE

You may end up needing to go to the bathroom somewhere that has only pay toilets.

## SCENT SPRAY

If you feel self-conscious about the smell—and let's be honest, few of us don't—pack a scent spray. The tricky thing is to avoid a chemical overlay of porta-potty-at-a-folk-festival smell, so a squirt of your favorite perfume usually isn't the best solution. For good results, use a dedicated product that works as an odor eliminator, rather than a cover-up. For example, products such as m9® spray by Hollister or any of the Poo-pourri® products work well in both close quarters and as room spray. There are also products such as YouGoGirl, a powder that you sprinkle on top of the water before you go. The powder turns in to foam, and not only does it provide a nice, fresh scent, it also muffles the sound *and* cleans the bowl. Superstar!

## BOOK/EREADER/MAGAZINE
Because you may be sitting in the bathroom for a while, and texting on the toilet is tacky. Multitask.

## PANTYLINERS
Periods aside, pantyliners are very useful if you have a small leak. Change often.

## TISSUES
In case you want to have a little cry, and believe me, there are times you will.

## SNACKS
Ideally, something you don't have to fiddle with a lot. It may sound excessive and counter-productive, but you may just be in the bathroom long enough to starve.

## DRINKS
Likewise, don't die of dehydration.

## PICTURES OF YOUR LOVED ONES
You may be on the toilet for so long you forget what they look like.

## ANTIBACTERIAL HAND WIPES/GEL
You never know if there will be soap. Plus, you won't feel so skeevy about eating that snack. DO NOT mix up with your baby wipes.

## NOTEPAD AND PAPER
Keep a diary, write a book, make lists (like this one). If you're feeling really rough, make a will.

## MOISTURIZER
You'll be washing your hands. A lot.

## TRICK SHOES
If you're very self-conscious (for example, if you are at work during a flare), bring an extra pair of shoes to the bathroom. Swap into them just before you let loose, then swap back to the originals when you leave. That way if anyone is nosy enough to look under the stall partition to try to identify the maker of that god-awful commotion, they'll never know it's you!

## A LIST INCLUDING YOUR CONDITION, MEDICATIONS, AND DOCTOR'S DETAILS
Just in case you pass out, are in an accident, or end up in prison. Having a list, or even a medical alert bracelet, is especially useful if you need to let someone know you are on steroids.

# SURVIVAL KIT TIPS

- Have several kits if you can. Keep one at work, one in the car, and one at your local pub. That way, you never have to worry about forgetting it.

- Keep everything together in a separate, dedicated bag. Don't just fill up your purse or man-bag with items.

- Keep your kit in an easily accessible location.

- If you don't want to carry full-sized products or buy travel-sized items, the dollar store is a great place to get travel sizes of bottles and containers.

- Keep anything that might spill or open in sealed, separate baggies within your kit.

# FISTULA SURVIVAL KIT

**WET WIPES**
Keep unscented skin wipes for sensitive skin or a soft cloth on hand to clean around your fistula.

**BARRIER CREAM**
If your skin is constantly irritated by discharge from your fistula, you may need to reapply barrier cream every time you go to the bathroom.

**ABSORPTION PAD**
If you use incontinence pads or sanitary pads, keep on hand a few more than you think you might need. Even if you don't normally use them, include some just in case.

**CHANGE OF UNDERWEAR**
You may never need them, but they're worth having for the peace of mind.

**DISPOSAL BAGS**
Dog poop bags, diaper sacks, or mini garbage bags are a discreet way to dispose of your dressings and used pads.

**HAND SANITIZER**
Just in case soap and water are not readily available.

**CHANGE OF DRESSING**
Pack several changes in case you have a sudden increase in discharge or are unable to access your home supply.

**MIRROR**
For fistulas in awkward places, a mirror will help you clean the site and change your dressing.

**SCISSORS**
Scissors are useful if you need to customize the size of your dressing.

## CUSHION

If you don't have room in your kit for a pillow, try an inflatable cushion that you can inflate or deflate as needed.

## OPTIONAL: ODOR-NEUTRALIZING SPRAY

If you are worried that your fistula discharge has an odor, carry a small bottle of odor spray.

# ADULT DIAPERS: NOT JUST A FETISH

Adult diapers get a lot of flack. Seen as the purview of the very young and the elderly, many teenagers and adults feel uncomfortable and even ashamed at the thought of having to wear a diaper during a flare-up of their ulcerative colitis. It's true that you can navigate these episodes without ever stepping into one. But honestly? Diapers can make your life during a flare a hell of a lot easier. I never thought of myself as someone who would ever wear diapers; I saw it as the surrender of the last tattered shreds of my feminine dignity.

One day I had the choice of either missing a special social occasion and staying home next to the toilet or putting on a diaper and going boldly. After much deliberation, I chose the latter. It was a revelation. I went out for the first time in months and *enjoyed* myself because I didn't have to worry about having an accident. Don't get me wrong. I did, several times—this was only two weeks after my j-pouch construction—but nobody noticed. Not a single person guessed that I was not only wearing a diaper, but had made good use of it. It actually seemed like people were much more concerned with what they were doing than what I may or may not have had on under my clothes. Funny that.

I only wish that I had gotten over the self-imposed stigma of wearing a diaper sooner. I feel no small regret when I think of all the things I missed doing when I had active ulcerative colitis and chose to stay home rather than wear something that no one else could see. And really, soiling the diaper wasn't a big deal. You make a mess, you clean it up, and you move on. Incontinence can be a fact of life when you have this condition, and there's no shame in it.

Besides, diapers are not for just the very young, old, infirm, or sexually experimental. They are also a staple of occupational wear. Want to know who else wears diapers?

- actors
- professional gamers
- surgeons and nurses
- astronauts
- scuba divers

- pilots
- political figures (during filibustering, for example)
- competitive weightlifters
- guards
- military personnel
- brides (yes, your wedding day is technically the first day of a new job)

So, you're in good company. If a diaper is good enough for a bride to wear on her wedding day, it's good enough for you.

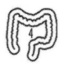

# 30,000 POUNDS OF BANANAS

## WHAT TO PUT IN YOUR MOUTH

### DIET DOS AND DON'TS

Once you've been diagnosed with ulcerative colitis, you'll find a lot of people suddenly have an opinion on what you should or shouldn't eat. A lot of this is down to people's ignorance of how colitis actually works. DIET DOES NOT CAUSE OR CURE ULCERATIVE COLITIS. Yes, diet can play a role in exacerbating or reducing your symptoms, and proper nutrition will obviously help you handle flares better when they do occur, but what you eat does not cause or cure your disease or its symptoms.

You will inevitably meet someone who claims they, or someone they know, have cured their ulcerative colitis by removing wheat from their diet, drinking goat wee, or only consuming air. These people did not have ulcerative colitis. What they likely had was a bad burrito and ennui. Ask these same people if they are self-diagnosed, and the answer will be yes. Unfortunately, the idea that your condition can be fixed by what you eat is propagated by an abundance of 'miracle' diet and recipe books and websites. While many of these diets are in fact good, healthy diets, they deceptively market themselves as a *cure* for ulcerative colitis. Sadly, many people with ulcerative colitis, or their loved ones, want this easy solution to be true. It isn't. If you're doing your best to eat properly and your ulcerative colitis still flares up, don't punish yourself for it. You've done as much as you can by eating well in the first place.

You'll also have more unsolicited advice regarding your diet from people who have no knowledge about your condition, but who feel perfectly competent telling you how to 'fix' it, than you'll have trips to the toilet. Initially, you may have the mindset of 'they're just trying to help,' but, really, they're not. If people were genuinely trying to give you helpful advice, they would take the time to understand what they were talking about. Offering advice about something they know nothing about isn't helpful—it's dismissive. Stop humoring them. One of the best ways to deal with this type of advice is to ask the person to explain exactly *how* not eating wheat will cure ulcerative colitis, and then sit back and watch them try to work it out. You may be waiting a long time, but it'll be worth it.

Your diet following your diagnosis should be aimed at:

- maintaining nourishment
- reducing symptoms, or at least, not aggravating them
- staying hydrated

When you're in remission, you can and should eat whatever you want. Try to keep your diet healthy and well-rounded, so that your body is in the best health it can be. Then, when you do have a flare, alter your diet accordingly. Don't be uptight about maintaining a strict diet. Get through the flare as best you can, then get back on track. There's no need to be more miserable than you already are. That said, don't use your flares as an excuse to eat nothing but cake either.

Luckily, you absorb most nutrients in your small bowel. If you lose weight during a flare, it's likely because you're eating less due to nausea, or because you know damn well that anything you put in your mouth will have to come out the other end. Many people reduce their caloric intake during a flare, however, eating less can make your flare worse since your body won't have the resources to cope.

You may also find that certain foods can make your symptoms worse. Although many of these foods seem to be universal irritants, some are unique to the individual. The best way to find out which foods do and don't work for you is to keep a food diary for the first few months after you're diagnosed, especially during a flare. Writing down what you ate can be helpful in identifying what you should or shouldn't be eating.

# DIET DOS FOR SURVIVING A FLARE

## TAKE A MULTI-VITAMIN (IF YOU'RE NOT TAKING ONE ALREADY)
Break the tablet in half, or use a gummy or liquid version to make sure it gets absorbed. Ensure the vitamin you choose has ample amounts of iron and calcium. If you are also taking sulfasalazine, take extra folic acid to ensure you absorb enough.

## DRINK LOTS OF WATER
Diarrhea will quickly dehydrate you. An electrolyte solution is a good choice if you are really suffering, but avoid those with too much sugar.

## PEEL FRUITS AND VEGETABLES
Fiber that is difficult to digest can irritate your colon during a flare, and the majority of fruit and vegetable fiber is in the peel.

## COOK FRUITS AND VEGETABLES
You don't need to cook them a lot, just enough to start breaking down the fiber.

## AVOID GASSY VEGETABLES
Like cabbage, beans, onions, radishes, cauliflower, and cucumber.

## EAT FOODS HIGH IN PROTEIN
You lose protein when you're bleeding, so increasing your protein intake will help you combat fatigue.

## KEEP EATING DAIRY
Many people think dairy is off-limits during a flare, but unless you're already lactose intolerant, or it makes you very gassy, include dairy. It's

a good source of calcium and protein.

## EAT FOODS HIGH IN IRON
Such as meat, eggs, and spinach. Adequate iron levels can help you avoid anemia.

## MAKE SMOOTHIES
Smoothies are a good option when you can't face eating solids. You can pack lots of protein, calcium, and other good stuff in them. They're also an easy way to include some fruit in your diet if you can't stomach it cooked.

## TAKE PROBIOTICS
There are a variety of prescription and over-the-counter probiotic live-culture yogurts and drinks available that may help replace good bacteria in your gut and improve your digestion.

## EAT SMALLER MEALS, MORE OFTEN
Grazing is a Good Thing.

## EAT FOODS THAT HAVE A BIT MORE SALT
With your colon inflamed, you may not be absorbing as much as you need. Don't overdo it.

## DRINK METAMUCIL®, OR OTHER BULKING AGENTS
The soluble fiber will give some soft bulk to your stool and help slow down your diarrhea without aggravating your colon.

## USE SEASONINGS
Spices are not the same as spicy. Your food doesn't have to be bland.

## EAT WHAT YOU WANT
If you're really struggling to eat, tempt yourself with whatever you can, even if it's junk. The important thing is to keep food going in—you can make up for it later.

## TAKE MEAL-REPLACEMENT DRINKS

If even the salty, processed nirvana of a Big Mac™ can't tempt you, you may have to resort to meal-replacement drinks. Yes, they taste like arse, but it is better than ending up in hospital where they'll force you to drink them through your nose.

# FLARE DIET DON'TS (OR AT THE VERY LEAST, USE CAUTION)

## DRINK ALCOHOL

It's tempting to drink yourself into oblivion until your flare is over, and while it will make you feel better in the short term, the sad truth is it will make your diarrhea even worse.

## DRINK CAFFEINE

Heart-breakingly, caffeine also increases diarrhea. You'll be amazed at the amount of liquid you're able to put out.

## DRINK CARBONATED DRINKS

Gas bubbles dilating your poor inflamed colon is painful and weirdly itchy.

## EAT A LOT (OR ANY) RAW FRUITS AND VEGETABLES

The raw fiber is difficult to digest and can increase bloating, gas, and cramps.

## EAT FOODS LIKE CORN, ONIONS, BEAN SPROUTS, AND MUSHROOMS

These foods are hard to digest properly even by "normal" people. Unless you really, really love them, give them a miss during your flare.

## DRIED FRUIT

Hard, shriveled fiber seems to really amp up the diarrhea.

## POPCORN, SEEDS, AND NUTS

Again, too much fiber.

## SPICY FOOD

It will burn even more on the way out.

## HIGH-FAT FOODS

This includes fried foods, fatty meats, and even peanut butter. Like sugar, alcohol, and too much fiber, fat can increase your diarrhea.

## BEANS

Too much fiber and gas-causing potential. If they happen to be your main source of protein, continue eating them, but have smaller portions and cook them well. Even better, puree them.

## SUGAR

Cutting back on sugar during a flare may interfere with your 'cake only' plan, but since sugar can increase both the cramping and diarrhea, it's probably best.

## USE A STRAW

Drinking through a straw can introduce air into your stomach, and a lot of it will have to rip through your colon to get out.

# IT'S BEETS!

Given your frequent brushes with intestinal and rectal bleeding, you can be forgiven for the surge of panic that rises upon the sight of a crimson-filled toilet bowl. But before you reach for the prednisone, ask yourself, "What did I eat today?"

As when you had a functioning colon, the color of what you put in your body influences the color of what comes out. The main difference now is that active disease in your colon will make any discoloration happen much quicker. Rather than seeing the result of those beets the next day, you may see them in a matter of hours—a much shorter time than you would expect. And in the early days when both paranoia and frequent bowel movements reign supreme, hysteria is a completely understandable reaction.

Be prepared to see carnage if you eat or drink any of the following:

- red wine
- beets
- licorice
- red Jell-o®
- tomato sauce
- any food with food coloring
- iron tablets
- spinach

# BULKING (YOUR STOOL, NOT YOUR MUSCLES)

When you have ulcerative colitis, the frequent, watery stools that have you constantly running for the bathroom are a nightmare. While you may find eating bran cereal is enough to slow things down, adding a bulking agent to your diet can thicken your stool, reduce the frequency with which you go, and absorb some of the digestive enzymes which damage your skin. Bulking agents are also an effective and natural alternative to antidiarrheal medications.

## TYPES OF BULKING AGENTS

### NATURAL PSYLLIUM FIBER
Sold commercially as Metamucil®, Konsyl®, Fiberall®, Isogel®, Fybogel®, Regulan® and Hydrocil®, psyllium (also known as ispaghula) is available as powdered drinks, capsules, bars, granules, or wafers.

### STERCULIA
Known as Normacol® in granular form.

### INULIN
The active fiber ingredient in FiberChoice® tablets.

### CELLULOSE
Sold as UniFiber®, cellulose is an insoluble fiber powder.

### METHYLCELLULOSE
A synthetic fiber usually sold as a powder or capsule under the name Citrucel®.

### POLYCARBOPHIL CALCIUM
Sold as Fibercon® and Mitrolan®, and available as a pill or chewable tablet.

## TIPS FOR USING BULKING AGENTS

- Start with a single dose a day and increase as needed. Do not exceed the recommended dosage.

- Take 30 minutes before eating to maximize absorption of digestive enzymes. Any later than that, and you'll reduce your appetite.

- Don't overdo it. If you feel constipated, are going to the bathroom much less than you normally would, or are having to strain, stop bulking until your movements loosen up.

- Take your dose without the recommended extra liquid, unless you feel you've over-bulked.

- Do not take if you suspect you have a blockage.

- Stop taking if you develop side effects including itching, severe gas, stomach or abdominal pain, nausea, or vomiting.

- You may find you are particularly gassy for the first few days, but this is usually temporary.

# PROBIOTICS

Probiotics are a frequent topic when you have inflammatory bowel disease. Their usefulness in helping relieve your symptoms is hotly debated—proponents hail them as a miracle cure while others insist there is no evidence they have any positive effect. The truth likely lies somewhere in the middle.

Because the exact cause of ulcerative colitis is not known, the specific role of probiotics and whether or not they help isn't clear. Like many natural treatments, probiotics seem to work very well for some people, not at all for others, and mostly, they seem to work for some people, some of the time. Clinical studies have yielded mixed results as to their effectiveness, yet all seem to agree that even though probiotics cannot prevent a flare of ulcerative colitis, or induce a patient into remission, they certainly pose no risk. In other words, probiotics won't cure you, but at worst, they may burn a hole in your wallet, and at best, they *may* help lessen the severity of your symptoms.

Probiotics can be prescribed by your doctor (VSL#3 is considered the gold standard), or you can buy both live or dormant strains from health food stores.

If you do decide to supplement your diet with probiotics, do it properly to increase your chance of success:

## DO YOUR RESEARCH
Probiotics can be very expensive, and not all formulations are covered by government healthcare or insurance. And because they are not considered to be a drug, the contents of most probiotics are not regulated.

## GET THE RIGHT ONE
Try to get a formulation that includes as many of the following as possible:
- *Bifidobacterium breve*
- *Bifidobacterium longum*
- *Bifidobacterium infantis*
- *Lactobacillus acidophilus*
- *Bactobacillus plantarum*

- *Lactobacillus paracasei*
- *Lactobacillus bulgaricus*
- *Streptococcus thermophilus*

## LIVE CULTURES ARE BEST

Live cultures are more expensive and need to be kept refrigerated, but they are also thought to be the most effective.

## KEEP A DIARY

Record how you feel daily for a few weeks before you begin taking probiotics, then for a few weeks after. Keeping track will make it easier for you to determine whether or not the probiotics are helping you.

## INFORM YOUR DOCTOR

Let your doctor know that you plan to take probiotics, and which ones you are going to use.

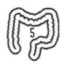

# THE HAND THAT FEEDS

## SURVIVING HEALTHCARE PROFESSIONALS

When you have ulcerative colitis, dealing with healthcare professionals can be frustrating. Issues you may encounter during your illness include:

### IGNORANCE OF YOUR CONDITION

Unless your family doctor or nurse is a specialist or has a lot of experience in gastroenterology, it probably took a long time for you to get properly diagnosed. Even with a diagnosis, you may find general physicians can be reluctant to deal with you when you're having a flare. Since it can take days, weeks, or even months to see a specialist, you may wait a long time to get treatment. Granted, most doctors are merely exercising prudence, especially when it comes to steroid therapy, but it can be difficult to accept this attitude when the doctor in question is hesitant to prescribe your needed medications even though they can see on your chart how you've been treated in the past.

### BEING DISMISSIVE OF YOUR CONDITION

Even dealing with a specialist can be upsetting at times; they likely treat patients whose conditions are more serious than yours, and you may feel that their level of concern is disproportionate to how awful you are feeling. Whether due to perspective on their part, or just a crappy bedside manner, don't take it personally. Try to keep your situation in perspective and remember that although they can have all the theoretical training in the world, unless they've experienced your condition for themselves, they can't truly understand it from your point of view.

## RIGIDITY OF TREATMENT PLANS

You've heard that anal bee stings are a cure for your colitis, and since it's a natural treatment, you would rather take on a bunch of bee pricks than subject yourself to a load of chemicals. You can't understand why your doctor doesn't think this is a good idea, and obviously, he's a big meanie for not exploring this with you.

There may be a time during your illness when you want to try alternative therapies that you *know* worked for other people—dear, sweet Internet, you'd never lie, would you? Many doctors will be open to your trying alternative treatments alongside your conventional ones if you can present it to them in a well-thought-out pitch. Bear in mind, however, that although they are not infallible, specialists have spent a lot of time and energy learning about your condition and how to treat it, and they prescribe certain medications because, in most cases, those treatments work. If nothing else, they don't want to look incompetent, so they are unlikely to make you take anything they don't genuinely think will help. Likewise, if they tell you that all you'll get from a bee sting is a fat ass, respect them enough to listen.

# TIPS FOR COPING WITH HEALTHCARE PROFESSIONALS

- Keep your expectations for care within your doctor's scope. They are not psychologists (unless they are). One professional deals with one set of issues.

- If you have chronic flares, ask your doctor for a standing prescription or extra refills so that you can treat yourself if necessary.

- Have your regular doctor recommend a course of treatment in your chart, in case you become ill in their absence.

- If your doctor has the personality and empathy of a wet fart, don't take it personally. It's tough being awesome all the time.

- If you feel you aren't being cared for properly, speak up. You may need to find another doctor.

- Be reasonable and realistic regarding the amount and type of care you expect.

- Accept that there might not be a perfect fix and that "well" is sometimes "well enough."

- Take as much responsibility for your own care as you can.

- Express yourself in a reasonable way. Being demanding or rude will get you nowhere. Understand that, galling as it may be, your doctor holds the power, and you need them on your side.

- A perky attitude can go far in helping you to receive better care. Don't be too perky, however, or the doctor may think there's nothing wrong with you.

- If you have to cry, cry pretty.

- You doctor is more likely to be flexible with your treatment if you're confident and capable in your self-care. Make sure you're knowledgeable, concise, and doing everything you can to keep yourself well outside of their help.

- Be willing to take advice, even if you're fairly certain it won't work for you. Your doctor or nurse will be more responsive if they feel you are trying.

- Take your medication. Yes, you may hate it or think you don't need it, but nothing will annoy a doctor more than if you refuse to follow your treatment plan and then bitch because you're not feeling well.

- That said, if you really don't agree with your doctor's plan, then don't follow it. Sometimes you do know better. Proceed with caution, however, because you may need to justify your decisions.

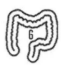

# GET UP, STAND UP
## EXERCISE AND ULCERATIVE COLITIS

## EXERCISE AND ULCERATIVE COLITIS

A hopeful question you may ask yourself now that you are afflicted with This Most Awful Disease is: "Do I still have to exercise?" Unfortunately, the answer is yes. And attending a seniors' armchair aerobics class or merely buying a Pilates DVD doesn't count.

Exercise is a Very Good Idea when you have ulcerative colitis, and many people with the disease are very physically active even during a flare. Like, triathlon active. Obviously, you don't have to go that far, but there is a good case for having a regular exercise regimen, even if only during remission. Exercise can help you cope with your ulcerative colitis by:

**KEEPING YOUR BODY IN GOOD SHAPE**
The healthier your body is, the more successfully you'll cope with flares. You may even find that exercise reduces the severity of your symptoms.

**GIVING YOU MORE ENERGY**
More energy will help you combat your fatigue.

**IMPROVING YOUR SELF-ESTEEM**
You may feel stinky but, by god, you'll be flexible.

## BOLSTERING YOUR MENTAL WELL-BEING

Burn the calories, eat twice as much cake.

## REDUCING STRESS

Ignoring, of course, the initial stress of having to get up and actually do it.

## AIDING DIGESTION

You'll need all the help you can get.

## KEEPING YOUR BONES STRONG

Use weight-bearing exercises to help counteract your steroids.

# TIPS FOR EXERCISING

For mere mortals, having ulcerative colitis means adjusting how you exercise, especially at the beginning of your illness (and if you're new to the whole 'exercise" thing) and during flares. To maximize your chances of starting and maintaining a successful and sustainable routine:

- Start slow and easy.

- Don't force it. Know when to quit—like during a flare, for example.

- Stay hydrated.

- Try low-impact exercises such as yoga, Pilates, swimming, golf, walking on the treadmill, or lifting weights.

- Avoid jarring movements such as running or aerobics, unless they are the aforementioned armchair aerobics. All that jostling can be painful if you're tender, and can also cause the dreaded anal leakage if you're in the middle of a flare.

- Practice pelvic floor exercises to improve your continence.

- Make sure you know exactly where the bathrooms are if you're exercising outdoors, or if you're having a flare, come prepared by wearing an adult diaper.

- If you don't want to wear a diaper, then a pantyliner or other undie protector should do.

- Bring your survival kit.

- Take an antidiarrheal and, of course, go to the bathroom before you begin.

- Apply moisture-barrier cream. If you're doing exercise right, chances are the inside of your butt cheeks is going to get nice and sweaty, so slather up to repel extra moisture and avoid chafing.

# PELVIC FLOOR EXERCISES

You likely consider anal continence a desirable commodity, and pelvic floor (Kegel) exercises can go a long way in helping you achieve it. As a bonus, doing Kegel exercises before and after your surgery also tightens your urinary and vaginal (or penal) muscles, bestowing you with the ultimate trifecta of desirability.

## HOW TO PERFORM THE KEGEL EXERCISE

1. Wait several weeks after your surgery before beginning or resuming the Kegels. Check with your doctor first to ensure you're good to go.

2. Locate the proper muscles by squeezing your sphincter as you do when you are desperately trying not to shart yourself. Clenching your cheeks is a bonus, not the focus.

3. At first, it may be easier to practice your Kegels while you are lying down. Lying down in bed with Netflix and a pound of chocolate makes it especially easy.

4. Tighten your pelvic floor muscles and hold for five seconds.

5. Relax for five seconds. Repeat.

6. Do four sets of five holds per day.

7. Keep breathing.

8. Work your way up to holding it for ten seconds, in sets of ten. Do this four times a day, forty clenches in all.

9. Once you become an expert at the basics, try practicing your Kegels without moving any muscles except your pelvic floor (no buttocks, thighs, abdomen, or face).

10. You can now perform your Kegels anywhere—at supper, at the movies, riding in your carriage—just remember to keep those face muscles neutral if you're in public.

11. Reap the benefit of pristine undies.

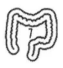

# LONG WAY FROM HOME
## TRAVEL AND SOCIAL EVENTS

## TRAVEL AND ULCERATIVE COLITIS

The idea of traveling with ulcerative colitis, especially during a flare, can be daunting. But with enough preparation, you should be able to travel as confidently as you did before.

### TIPS FOR SUCCESSFUL TRAVEL

**BEFORE YOU GO**

- Learn your destination's local language for directions to the bathroom.

- Get extra refills of your prescriptions, and copy your prescription notes to take through security.

- Ensure you're aware of the bathroom situation in the country you're visiting. Although many countries have Western-style toilets, going off the beaten track can mean squat toilets. Make sure that you feel confident using one beforehand by practicing with a bucket. Some countries provide water hose attachments rather than toilet paper—you may find this system actually works better than Western-style, especially if your skin is tender from a flare.

Also be aware that some countries do not have a lot of public bathrooms available.

- If available, download the bathroom locator app for that country.

- Accept that your backpacking days may be over, unless you are confident with your state of remission.

- Don't scrimp or lie on your medical insurance.

- Note the location of local hospitals.

- Get a medic alert bracelet indicating that you have ulcerative colitis, especially if you are on steroids at the time of travel.

## ON THE PLANE

- Book an aisle seat, and near the toilet if you can. Most airline companies and agents are very accommodating if you explain your situation.

- Buy or bring your own snacks, since you never know what the airline will be serving, and special diets aren't available on all flights. A medical note from your doctor can help with security if necessary.

- Take your full set of prescription medications on the flight with you, and keep another set in your check-in luggage so you'll be covered if one set gets lost.

- Bring your own toilet paper and wipes. The economy toilet paper on most planes is worse than in prison.

- Gravol® or other anti-nausea medication can be useful if you're anxious about flying during a flare; it can make you sleepy and may also constipate you slightly.

- Bring a change of clothes in case of accidents.

- Wear an adult diaper if you're having a flare, just to be on the safe side. You never know how long you may have to wait for the bathroom—people are often not as accommodating in the air as they are on the ground.

- Take a blanket or shawl. Apparently you have to pay extra to both fly and be warm.

- Buy water after you go through security. Stay hydrated. An electrolyte power drink is also a good idea, but avoid trying to bring a home-packaged powder through security.

- Bring a few doses of a bulking agent, just in case you're on a long-haul and things get loose.

- Take toilet seat covers and antibacterial hand wash. Other people are gross.

## IN THE CAR

- Map out the bathrooms en route.

- Pack a porta-potty, such as those used for camping and hunting.

- Stay hydrated, but limit your intake if you know you might not be able to make a pit-stop.

- Diapers, diapers, diapers!

- Go whenever and wherever you have a chance, even if you don't really have to go.

- Keep your survival kit within easy reach.

## ONCE YOU'RE THERE

- Be adventurous with what you eat (after all, you're on holiday), but not too adventurous. When in doubt, go for safe foods—anything familiar and well-cooked.

- Try to avoid food poisoning at all costs. Avoid buffets, and use your judgment when buying from street vendors. If in doubt, pack snacks.

- Be extra careful with water hygiene, including ice cubes. Contaminated water is the easiest way to get traveler's diarrhea.

- Don't stress. You can do that at home.

- Keep copies of your documents on hand at all times, including a description of your condition, a list of your medications, your doctor's name and phone number, and your insurance details.

- Keep change on you at all times for pay toilets.

- Take your survival kit, or a pared-down version, everywhere.

# SOCIAL EVENTS

When you're ill with a chronic condition—especially one that causes rampant diarrhea—socializing is not as straightforward as it once was. With a little foresight and planning, however, it can still be just as fun.

## TIPS FOR STRESS-FREE SOCIALIZING DURING A FLARE

- Bring your survival kit. If your kit is large, pare it down to the bare essentials or carry travel sizes.

- Do a bathroom reconnaissance when you arrive. Know where the bathrooms are so you don't have to run around frantically looking for them when you do actually need to go.

- If you are at a restaurant, don't make a big production about what you can and can't eat. If you can't eat the mushrooms, fine. You don't have to order them. Nor do you have to explain to everyone WHY you can't order them. Just choose something else.

- If you're having a meal at someone's house, let your host know ahead of time what you can't eat. Otherwise you risk making them feel awkward when you can't eat what they're serving.

- Eat slow, small, and what you know. Don't take risks just because it's a special occasion.

- Don't get wasted. Being blind drunk can increase your risk of accidents.

- Don't talk about your illness all night. The whole point of going out is that everyone enjoys themselves. Don't ruin it by boring everyone to death. If somebody asks, fine. But keep it brief and clean.

- Always have an exit strategy. If the people you're with know about your condition, you don't need to make excuses—just tell them you don't feel well and leave. If they're unaware of your illness, decide in advance how much (or little) you want to tell them, or just say you have a headache.

- If you have an accident while you are out, deal with it, and try not to let it ruin your night. Having an accident in public can be daunting, but if you're prepared, you can sort it out quickly. Don't let the fear of accidents at any stage of your illness keep you from going out. If you're in the middle of a bad flare, take preemptive action by wearing a diaper.

- Get your outfit ready the day before, plus a back-up. This way you will not be stressing at the last minute.

- If you are obligated to attend a social event while you have a flare, standing around, walking, or dancing may not be activities that you feel capable of doing. Just sit at your table and let people come to you. You'll look much cooler that way, anyway.

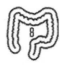

# SHAKE IT OUT

## THE EMOTIONAL IMPACT OF ULCERATIVE COLITIS

## THE EMOTIONAL IMPACT OF ULCERATIVE COLITIS AND HOW TO COPE

At first, many people with ulcerative colitis are happy just to have a diagnosis and begin treatment. In fact, the reality of your situation may not hit you until your next flare, which could be weeks, months, or even years down the road. Like the physical manifestations of the disease, most people seem to experience similar emotional reactions to their condition. Understandably, these reactions are remarkably like the stages of grief. You are dealing with a significant loss: of yourself as you were, and of the course of your life as you understood and planned it. A loss of this kind is no small thing, but it often seems that its impact is underestimated not only by the person with ulcerative colitis, but also by their loved ones, and by the community at large. Even many health care providers don't fully appreciate the psychological effects of living daily with the disease once the initial crisis and diagnosis are over. You may find that you experience some or all of the following feelings:

**DENIAL**
After the relief of diagnosis, you may feel a sense of denial. You may:

- Refuse to accept that you have ulcerative colitis. Some

people cling to the idea that they have only a severe form of IBS.

- Reject the idea that you will have to take medication for the rest of your life to keep the disease under control.
- Ignore the extent to which ulcerative colitis will impact your quality of life, or underestimate how much the disease will affect your everyday routine. Many of us seem to be guilty of harboring a bizarre belief that we are special, and somehow the condition will not affect us as much as the next person.
- *Over*estimate the extent to which ulcerative colitis will impact your quality of life.

## HELPLESSNESS

Most people find a lack of control difficult to deal with, and ulcerative colitis provides chaos in abundance. You may:

- Feel out of control. Ulcerative colitis is a disease that has no prevention and no cure. Even removing your colon is only a partial solution.
- Realize there is nothing you can do to prevent a flare from eventually happening. No matter how good your diet is, how much you exercise, or how stress-free your life is, your illness will eventually trigger a flare.
- Feel helpless at the lack of control over the extent of your flares—your symptoms may be mild, or they may be severe.
- Find you often cannot control your symptoms even when you're in remission, such as fatigue or the side-effects of your medication. You never really know how you will feel day-to-day.

## FEAR

Fear is another significant aspect of ulcerative colitis. The disease can be a big shadow to live under, and you may feel you are constantly holding your breath and waiting for your condition to get worse. Much of the fear associated with ulcerative colitis can surround your lifelong prospects. You may:

- Feel anxious about your long-term prognosis, such as whether you will need to have surgery, or whether you will develop colon cancer.
- Worry about the continuing effects of your medications.
- Be concerned about how the disease and your symptoms will affect your career, and how it will impact your relationships with partners, family, and friends.
- Find that you have to re-evaluate your plans for the future.
- Fear that your basic quality of everyday life will deteriorate to the point that you will find it unbearable.

## NEGATIVE BODY IMAGE

You may find that your body image takes a beating; nothing lowers self-esteem like rampant diarrhea. You may:

- Feel extra self-conscious about your bodily functions, especially if you are a person who already finds it difficult to work-poop.
- Feel bloated and gross. The combination of medication side-effects and the ulcerative colitis itself create a perfect storm of generally feeling like crap.
- Feel stinky. Even if people tell you that you don't smell, you may feel like there is a constant stink-cloud hovering over you.
- Feel like never letting anyone see you naked ever again. Unlike nymphomania, ulcerative colitis feels like one of the least sexy diseases ever.

## ANGER AND FRUSTRATION

Anger seems to be another prevalent emotion when coping with ulcerative colitis. As if you didn't already have enough stuff to be pissed off about, what with periods, the remake of the *Wicker Man*, and the fact that Cranberry Ginger Ale® is sold only at Christmas, you may:

- Be angry that the disease happened to you in the first place.
- Resent that you have to have treatment for the rest of your

life or face complicated surgery.

- Feel like your body is no longer your own, as it is continually subjected to a host of invasive and often embarrassing procedures.
- Be frustrated that your quality of life and your ability to function are compromised, and that your best efforts to overcome this may, at times, fail.
- Feel defeated by the general ignorance surrounding ulcerative colitis which, given its nature and our feelings about bodily functions, is not openly discussed.

## DEPRESSION

All of these feelings can build high levels of stress and anxiety, which can ultimately lead to depression. If you've suffered from depression even before you developed ulcerative colitis, the emotional impact of the condition can be especially catastrophic. Signs you may be becoming depressed include:

- Being unwilling or unable to care for yourself properly.
- Finding it difficult to speak to anyone about what you are feeling, or to seek help.
- Being unable to cope with things you would have had no trouble with before.
- Over or underreacting to situations.
- Withdrawing from your relationships and support network.
- Feeling suicidal.

## COPING WITH THE EMOTIONAL IMPACT OF ULCERATIVE COLITIS: METHODS, PROS, AND CONS

### GETTING ON WITH IT

(Ulcerative colitis? Ha! You laugh in the face of ulcerative colitis. It's all just a bit inconvenient, really.)

**Pros:**

- Much more convenient and comfortable for those around you.
- Mad props; everybody loves a hero.
- Can actually take you pretty far.
- As Kurt Vonnegut said: "One of the most impressive ways to tell your war story is to refuse to tell it, you know. Civilians would then have to imagine all kinds of deeds of derring-do."

**Cons:**

- When you finally get overwhelmed and break down, and you will, you will go down hard.
- Martyrdom can be addictive, and can eventually put your quality of life, and even your life itself, at risk.
- People will assume that you're fine, which can make it difficult for them to understand when you're suddenly not.
- Contributes to misunderstanding the disease's impact, both at your personal level and as part of the bigger picture.

## TALKING TO FRIENDS AND FAMILY
(Sometimes at great length . . . )

**Pros:**

- Can be very helpful and therapeutic.
- Having people understand your issues and limitations even a little can make living with ulcerative colitis easier.
- Other people often feel better if they know where things stand.

**Cons:**

- Some people just don't want to know. It may be that they're just not interested, or that they are uncomfortable with the subject matter, because hmygoodpoopissogross.
- You can over-explain or over-share, which can make people uncomfortable. Keep it clean and concise.
- You can overburden people if you talk about your illness too much, even those who are interested. People are sympathetic to a point. Understand that it's your issue, not

theirs. Constantly discussing it will make you boring, and eventually, even your mother will begin to avoid you.

## RESEARCHING YOUR ILLNESS
(Know *everything* there is to know.)

**Pros:**
- Can make you feel more prepared—often this will help you to cope better.
- Can increase your confidence.
- Can put your condition in perspective.
- Can help you make informed choices.

**Cons:**
- Sometimes you can know too much. For example, the long-term risks of the medication you take and your long-term prognosis are things that you have very little control over. Risk is attached to everything in life, and focusing on things that may (or may not) happen can increase your stress levels and aggravate your illness.
- Can lead to obsession. Unless you are planning to become a paid specialist in the field, learn what you need to know, then move on. Go out and live. None of that knowledge will help you in the zombie apocalypse, anyway.

## PARTICIPATING IN ONLINE FORUMS
(Drop in, drop out, lurk, or chat—just don't feed the trolls.)

**Pros:**
- Forums can be helpful. It can be reassuring to speak to people in a similar situation and to share experiences.
- There are some wonderful, supportive people in forums who are happy to help with any support you might need.
- Forums can be a great source of practical advice on all aspects of the disease, especially if you are experiencing complications.
- If you are having a particular problem, chances are very good that someone else in a forum has had, or is having, it

as well.

- You can drop in and out of forums as you wish.

**Cons:**

- Forums can be an insidious black hole of self-pity.
- Forums can have a strange culture of competition over who has it worse and they may make you feel as though your legitimate concerns are invalid and should be dismissed.
- Forums can present a skewed picture of ulcerative colitis, especially if you're a newbie. Keep in mind that many people use forums only when they are struggling, so people who are successfully coping tend to be underrepresented. This disproportionate representation can make your situation seem grimmer that it actually may be.

## READING PERSONAL BLOGS

(An individual's account of their experience, from diagnosis to present-day.)

**Pros:**

- You get a comprehensive view of what life can be like with ulcerative colitis, including the ups as well as the downs.
- Personal blogs can be a great source of inspiration.

**Cons:**

- Each blog represents only a single person's experience, and you may want specific information that isn't covered by that particular blog.

## ATTENDING SUPPORT GROUPS

(Like the *Breakfast Club*: nobody really wants to be there, but it may just change your life.)

**Pros:**

- The same as the forums, but without many of the cons.
- You have to get up off your ass and go to meetings. Gets you out and about, if only briefly.
- Meetings can be quite fun, and you might even make some

friends.

- What is the point of being in an exclusive club if you don't go to meetings?
- Often the food is quite good.

**Cons:**

- There may not be a support group where you live. If not, see if there is any local interest and then start your own. To get people to attend, promise cake or puppies.
- As with forums, there is sometimes competition over who has it the hardest. Don't let other people diminish your struggle. For all you know, they may just be trying to get extra cake.
- There is the possibility of emotional pirates, who can be difficult to get away from in a face-to-face situation. Some extremely needy person may attach themselves to you and not let go. And, of course, being a nice person, you will politely let them strangle you—this can hamper your ability to cope. Your needs come first, so carry a crowbar. Harsh, but this *is* a matter of survival.

## SEEKING PROFESSIONAL HELP

(For those times when it all becomes too much.)

**Pros:**

- Can give you an extra level of support.
- Can evaluate you for an anti-depressant or anti-anxiety medication if you need it, and many people do.
- Talking to someone you don't know personally can help you explore your feelings in a way that might not be possible with your friends and family. That urge to strangle your partner after the hundreth poop joke? Best not mention that to *them*.
- Can help you devise personalized coping strategies.

**Cons:**

- If your therapist does not commonly treat patients with chronic illness, it may be difficult for them to appreciate its impact on you.

- Some people feel there's a stigma, both on their part and from other people, attached both to depression and to seeking professional help, especially for a condition many people consider "just diarrhea."

# RELATIONSHIPS AND ULCERATIVE COLITIS

Chronic illness impacts relationships. Regardless of the severity of your ulcerative colitis, the dynamics of your relationships with your spouse, family, friends, and co-workers will change and influence your relationship in both negative and positive ways.

## NEGATIVE EFFECTS ON YOUR RELATIONSHIPS

### PEOPLE UNDERESTIMATE THE EFFECTS OF THE DISEASE

Ulcerative colitis is an 'invisible' illness. There are few external symptoms of the disease, even when you are in the midst of a flare. You will often *look* fine, and so unless you invite people into the bathroom with you, they'll assume that you *are* fine. Consequently, people can become resentful if they think you're using your diagnosis as an excuse not to engage in certain activities, such as work or social obligations.

### PEOPLE OVERESTIMATE THE EFFECTS OF THE DISEASE

Parents, spouses, and children may become overprotective of you, which can create a difficult situation. You may feel resentful at being treated like a child and feel like your independence is restricted. It can also be tempting to take advantage of people's willingness to do things for you, even when you are perfectly capable of doing them for yourself.

### LOVED ONES (AND STRANGERS) TRY TO BECOME OVERLY INVOLVED IN YOUR CARE

They may spend hours researching ways to make you feel better or even "cure" you, and may subsequently feel hurt or see you as combative when you don't submit to their carefully-researched regimen of drinking a pint of aloe vera juice every morning.

## YOUR LOVED ONES FEEL ANGRY AND SCARED ABOUT WHAT IS HAPPENING TO YOU, AND WORRY ABOUT WHAT WILL HAPPEN IN THE FUTURE.

Reassuring them can be difficult, especially during the times when you are obviously unwell.

## FAMILY OR FRIENDS FEEL ANGRY OR RESENTFUL

Some people may feel jealous, not because they want a disease, although this can happen as well, but because of the attention you receive.

## YOUR COWORKERS START TO HATE YOU

A flare can progress so quickly that there will be times when you seem fine one day and then are off work the next, and this can be difficult for coworkers to understand. Some may think that your frequent trips to the toilet are a way of avoiding work, or a method of manipulating a lighter workload. And if you actually *do* have to reduce your workload, even periodically, your coworkers can become resentful of what they perceive as your inability to do your job properly and "carry your weight."

## PEOPLE TRY TO TAKE ADVANTAGE OF YOU AND YOUR SITUATION

Some people may consider you in a weakened state and may attempt to usurp certain positions you hold, such as at work or within personal relationships.

## YOUR MARRIAGE OR PARTNERSHIP MAY BECOME STRAINED

Ulcerative colitis seems to polarize marriages. At times, you will become more physically, emotionally, and even financially dependent on your spouse, and there will likely be a change in physical intimacy. You may find these changes bring a new bond of strength to your relationship; however, you may also find your spouse simply can't cope.

# POSITIVE EFFECTS ON YOUR RELATIONSHIPS

## STRENGTHENS YOUR MARRIAGE OR RELATIONSHIP

Your spouse and parents may occasionally become your caregiver. Many people find that their loved ones relish the role, as it allows them to help you and makes them feel more connected to you.

## HELPS CHILDREN LEARN TO NURTURE

It is important for children to learn how to cope with other people's vulnerability in a caring and helpful way. It can also give them feelings of confidence and positive self-esteem if they feel needed and can help you.

## BRINGS OUT THE BEST IN PEOPLE

You may be pleasantly surprised at how much people care. You may find that people are very supportive and want to take part in activities to raise awareness about your condition, such as sponsored walks and bake sales. Especially bake sales. People *love* bake sales.

## PREVENTS YOU AND YOUR LOVED ONES FROM TAKING YOUR RELATIONSHIP FOR GRANTED

Serious illness can make people stop and think about the person involved and how their lives would be affected if that person wasn't there. You may find that both you and your loved ones want to affirm your relationships and make more of an effort to show how much you value each other.

## HELPS OTHERS CONFIDE IN YOU

You may find that people are more willing to discuss their own issues with you, especially if those issues are related to their health.

# COPING WITH THE CHANGES IN YOUR RELATIONSHIPS

## ANSWER PEOPLE'S QUESTIONS THE BEST YOU CAN

Some of these questions will seem ignorant to you, but not knowing something is the definition of ignorance. Most people who ask you questions are genuinely interested but don't have the time to research something that doesn't directly affect them.

## ACCEPT THAT NOT EVERYONE HAS THE TIME, THE PATIENCE, OR THE SYMPATHY TO LEARN ABOUT YOUR ILLNESS

It can be devastating to realize this, especially if it the person is someone close to you. Even though it is personal, don't take it personally.

## BE AS INDEPENDENT AS YOU CAN, BUT RECOGNIZE WHEN YOU NEED HELP AND ASK FOR IT

People will better understand what you are going through if you include them. Also, if you don't ask for help when you are obviously struggling, you risk people thinking that you're trying to be a martyr.

## BE CLEAR AND FIRM (BUT DIPLOMATIC) ABOUT WHAT YOU NEED AND WHAT YOU DON'T

Then everyone, including you, knows where they stand.

## DON'T LET YOUR ILLNESS DEFINE YOU

The more you do, the more severely your relationships will be affected. Even though you're sick, you still have to put effort into your relationships.

## CONSIDER WHETHER YOUR CURRENT EMPLOYMENT IS GOING TO WORK FOR YOU

Be realistic. If you feel that you may not be able to carry out your duties adequately, you may have to reconsider your career.

## ACCEPT THAT SOME RELATIONSHIPS, WHETHER THEY BE PARTNERS, FAMILY, OR FRIENDS, ARE NOT WORTH HAVING

There will be some people who simply cannot cope with your illness, often because they lack the empathy to understand your condition beyond its inconvenience to them. Some people are just knobs like that. Treat yo'self and get rid.

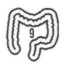

# AFTERNOON DELIGHT

## SEX, PREGNANCY, AND ULCERATIVE COLITIS

## SEX AND ULCERATIVE COLITIS

Although you probably won't feel much like having sex during a flare—unless the person is really cute or it's their birthday—you may find that you experience some physical and emotional changes in regards to your sexuality, even while you are in remission.

### PHYSICAL CHANGES AND ISSUES

#### REDUCED LIBIDO
Due to the effects of your medication, a recent flare-up, or even general pain and fatigue, you may find that you're just not as up for it as you were before.

#### INCONTINENCE
You may find you have some incontinence during sex. Leakage usually only occurs during a flare.

#### PAIN
You may find penetration uncomfortable or even painful. Pain can be due to a fistula, an abscess, or an infection, or you may have abdominal tenderness that becomes painful when under pressure. If you are having, or are about to have a flare, you may have rectal and/or

perianal pain.

## NAUSEA
You may find energetic movement makes you nauseous. Of course, depending on what kind of sex you have, this may not be a problem.

## STIFFNESS
Joint pain may mean you're not as limber as you once were.

## TENESMUS
You may suddenly feel the urge to go to the bathroom.

# EMOTIONAL CHANGES AND ISSUES

You may:

- Feel awkward about explaining your condition to new partners, especially if they are unfamiliar with the disease or have a limited understanding of it.
- Feel embarrassed about what your partner may think of your condition, and worried they might not find you attractive because of it.
- Feel like you're not your normal self physically, and your confidence may be compromised.
- Be worried about leakage, pain, odor, needing to go to the toilet, or even about the impact on the relationship if you turn down sex.
- Just not be interested. Sex may not be a priority for you—being constantly probed for medical purposes may put you off recreational probing.

# TIPS FOR SEX WITH ULCERATIVE COLITIS

- Avoid sex during a flare, unless you're really into it.

- Do not feel guilty for not wanting to have sex.

- Try to schedule windows for "spontaneous" sex, for example, at those times of day when you are feeling less tired.

- Keep in mind that your partner does not see you the way you feel. You may feel unattractive; they probably think you're hot. (The pale, slightly green complexion was a huge hit in the Victorian times.)

- Go to the bathroom before engaging.

- Light a few scented candles for your own peace of mind.

- Make yourself feel sexy, in all the same ways that you did before your diagnosis.

- Foreplay is even more essential.

- Use lubrication if penetration is uncomfortable at first.

- Try different positions to find the one that is the most comfortable.

- Go slow.

- Avoid penetration if it's too painful—there's lots of other stuff you can do. (Google it.)

- DO NOT use a suppository beforehand.

- Avoid any butt-play, if that area is sensitive or tender.

- If you suddenly feel the urge to the toilet during sex, GO. Do not try to hold it in. Yes, stopping sex so you can use the toilet may ruin the mood, but so will pooping on someone else's naughty bits.

- Reassure your partner that you are fine and are enjoying yourself.

- Be positive. It's much, much sexier than a grimace.

- Persevere! That said, know when to give up and cuddle.

# PREGNANCY AND ULCERATIVE COLITIS

Some good news about ulcerative colitis is that your fertility usually remains unaffected, and although you may have an increased risk of complications during your pregnancy, most women with ulcerative colitis have normal pregnancies and healthy babies. Associated risk of miscarriage or stillbirth comes from the effect of the disease on *you*, not the ulcerative colitis itself. The healthier you are, the lower your risk for complications.

Most doctors recommend trying to get pregnant only when you are in remission, since many women who become pregnant during a flare continue to have active disease during their pregnancy. Active colitis impacts the quality of your health and can subsequently increase the risk of complications such as miscarriage, low birth weight, and premature birth. A common recommendation is for you to be in a remission state for at least three months prior to conception, but for many women, this is not realistic.

## TIPS FOR COPING WITH PREGNANCY AND ULCERATIVE COLITIS

### BEFORE PREGNANCY

- If you're taking methotrexate, stop taking it three to six months before you begin trying to conceive. Methotrexate has been identified as increasing the risk of birth defects and spontaneous abortion, nor is it safe while you are pregnant or breastfeeding.
- Ensure your diet is well-balanced.
- Be as physically fit as possible.
- Have your folic acid levels tested and make sure that you are supplementing your diet with adequate amounts. Certain medications, such as sulfasalazine, will lower your levels of folic acid by inhibiting its absorption.
- Ensure your iron levels are sufficient, especially if you are prone to anemia.

- Ideally, you should be off steroids at the time of conception.

## DURING PREGNANCY

- Hemorrhoids may be worse, so stock up on cream.
- Even if you're in remission at the time of conception, your pregnancy may still be considered high-risk for complications. You might be placed under the care of both a gastroenterologist and an obstetrician for the duration of your pregnancy, especially if it's your first.
- Continue to eat the best diet you can manage. Just like pregnant women without ulcerative colitis, the healthier you are, the better the chance your baby will be too.
- Check with your doctor to determine which of your medications you can continue taking.
  According to the Crohn's and Colitis Foundation of America, the associated risks of harming your baby are generally considered to be:

**Aminosalicylates:** no known risk.
**Corticosteroids:** low risk.
**Immunomodulators:** low, with the exception of methotrexate.
**Biologics:** low risk in early to mid-pregnancy.
**Antibiotics:** variable risk. Use only if the benefit outweighs the risk.

**Always check with your doctor before starting or stopping any medications.**

## GIVING BIRTH

- Unless you have an abscess or a fistula, you should be able to give birth as you would have done had you not had ulcerative colitis.

## AFTER BIRTH

- Some women find they experience a flare in the days directly after delivery.
- Ulcerative colitis does not influence breastfeeding, although you will have to continue to take only advised medications.

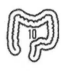

# PAJAMAS ALL DAY

## WHAT TO WEAR DURING A FLARE

### FLARE FASHION DOS

**HAVE TWO WARDROBES: ONE FOR REMISSION AND ONE FOR FLARES**
Two sets of clothes will make life easier. One day you'll fit into your skinny jeans, the next you won't.

**RUNNING SHOES**
Because you may have to run.

**STRETCH DENIM AND LEGGINGS**
Will streamline bloat and make you more aerodynamic as you race to the toilet. Just make sure they're not too tight.

**MATERNITY PANTS AND ELASTIC WAISTS**
You'll wish you hadn't waited until you were actually pregnant to wear these. Heaven.

**LOWRIDERS**
Low waistbands can be a bit of love/hate situation. They may give your tender abdomen plenty of room to breathe, but when you're bloated, you'll end up with a muffin top.

**DIAPERS**
Let go of your inhibitions and embrace them if you need them. The

peace of mind is invaluable. Plus, everyone knows that Japan is one of the most style-forward countries in the world, and diapers are big business there.

## TAILORED DRESSES
Especially tea dresses, swing dresses, or anything else that flares at the waist—they're comfortable, and flatter every figure.

## CLEAVAGE-ENHANCING TOPS
If you're going to gain steroid weight, you may as well own it.

## PATTERNED CLOTHING
Patterns are great if you're feeling self-conscious about weight fluctuations. Also good if you're worried people can see your diaper.

## SWEATPANTS/ LOUNGE PANTS
Soft, comfortable, and forgiving. Use responsibly. There is a fine line between causal chic and giving up. Stay classy.

## JEWELRY, MANICURES, PEDICURES, MAKE-UP
They may say you can't polish a turd, but you can sure make it sparkle.

# FLARE FASHION DON'TS

## WEAR PLAYSUITS, PANTSUITS, OR ONESIES
You may look cute as all hell, but you might need to get your pants down quickly. If your outfit comes off from the top down, there will be a significant time delay until you can drop trou, not to mention the added risk of brushing the top of your outfit against the toilet and floor.

## WEAR HEELS
Unless you can Bryce Dallas Howard that shit, save yourself the agony.

## WEAR WHITE BOTTOMS
Of any kind. Ever. Why tempt fate?

## SWEATPANTS WITH A SLOGAN SCRAWLED OVER THE ASS

Unless it says 'Hot Mess' or 'Attention Whore.' This is just general advice, by the way, nothing to do with ulcerative colitis.

## POLYESTER UNDERWEAR

The moistness. The chafing. The smell of despair.

## TIGHT CLOTHES

Both your tender, bloated gut and your self-esteem will thank you.

# A WORD ABOUT ULCERATIVE COLITIS AND HAIR

It seems many people who undergo a life-changing experience develop an overwhelming desire to get a drastic haircut. Break-ups, childbirth, loss: there is something about realizing the impermanence of life that makes you realize your hairstyle at that particular moment is not the one you want to be buried in.

I have been through this ritual a number of times. After my first major stay in the hospital when I was diagnosed, I chopped my long hair into what I thought was a cute, playful bob. It was a huge mistake. Not getting a haircut, but that *particular* haircut. It turns out that a chin-length, rounded bob + steroids = moon face-bobble-head doll, and not in a cute way. Luckily for me, the steroids made most of my hair fall out shortly after.

I then discovered wigs—beautiful, wonderful wigs. Long, black, and silky wigs; sleek, platinum bobs; sassy, red, feathered layers. I'm sure it was obvious to everyone that those wigs were not my real hair—they were pretty damn fabulous—but I didn't care. God, I loved those wigs. Unfortunately, so did the cat.

After my second long hospital stay, I shaved my hair into a 'Chelsea,' which is such a strong haircut that no one notices the size of your face. I then managed to overcome the makeover urge after each of my three surgeries, but finally broke and shaved one half of my head soon after my son was born. When he wore his first "big boy" shirt with actual buttons, I shaved the other side. When he got his first teeth, I got a dip-dye.

I can only speculate on my particular reasons for both the need for constantly evolving hair and its effect on me. That first haircut, even as awful as it was, gave me a sense of control over something at a time when so much of my life was out of my hands. Changing the way I looked on the outside allowed me to grieve, and it helped me to accept the changes that were happening on the inside—the new person I was becoming. It was also a result of plain old rebellion. (Screw you, body, I'll show you who's driving this bus.)

The second time, it wasn't so much about becoming a new me. I had accepted that my life had forever changed, and what I needed then was a badge of badassery to help keep me moving forward. I wanted to look as fierce on the outside as I felt on the inside. That hair shifted my focus away from my illness and encouraged me to progress.

Sporting a new hairstyle in general—and those wigs in particular—was also a way for me to claw back my femininity. I had never thought of myself a vain person until I woke up one morning with my hair festooning my shoulders like the world's most pathetic stole. It felt like a kick in the teeth after everything I had just gone through, and how unattractive I already felt. There was something about my hair being the last bastion of my womanhood when the rest of my body had gone to pot. The worst part was when people tried to be nice about it. "Your hair is thinning? I hadn't noticed. I thought comb-overs were the new thing." Those wigs gave me back a sense of femininity and fun that, at the time, was crucial to my sense of well-being and recovery. I continued to wear them occasionally even after my hair grew back—which it did, curly.

Other times, radically changing my hair gave me a visible symbol of the choice I had made between wallow or fight. Now every time I look in the mirror, I see a warrior, and my choice is reaffirmed. It may sound incredibly superficial, but for me, it works, and I am a better mother and stronger person for it.

I don't know if this approach would work for everyone. I personally find the process cathartic and empowering. And if it goes horribly wrong, who cares? Unlike your colon, your hair will grow back.

# TIPS FOR ULCERATIVE COLITIS AND HAIR

- Because of your medications and stress, your hair may fall out. Look at it as an opportunity to try new looks.

- Your hair, if it does fall out, may grow back curly. Or, if it is curly, it may grow back straight.

- Changing your hair is something you can control. It may be a small victory, but it's a victory nonetheless.

- A new hairstyle may help you symbolically start your "new" life.

- Regret is for the things you don't do. Hair will grow back.

- Your new style can be as subtle or drastic as you like. You don't have to shave your head. You can get just a stripe of color, anything.

- If you are feeling especially vulnerable, don't get a drastic cut. There is a good chance it will make you feel even worse. Start small.

- If the result is awful, at least it will shift both your and other people's attention away from your illness, however briefly.

- If you are on steroids and have a moon-face, avoid a chin-length or above-chin bob, short curly hair, rounded hairstyles, hairstyles that flare at the sides, heavy straight-across blunt bangs, and center parts at all costs. Height and length are Very Good Things.

- Wigs are GLORIOUS.

# ASSHOLES EVERYWHERE
## THE PEOPLE YOU'LL MEET

Once you become the proud owner of an invisible chronic illness, you will be (un)pleasantly surprised by how many ignorant assholes worm their way out of the woodwork. Most of these queries are from well-meaning people, but in the moment of contact, you'll find that rationalization gives you surprisingly little comfort.

Funnily enough, having a chronic illness may not stop you being one or two of these people yourself. The following are the most common people you will meet, so prepare yourself. And if you don't have a chronic illness yourself, but know someone that does (and that's why you're reading this book), don't be these people. Do all of us sickies a solid and learn how to use Google.

### THE "REALLY? YOU'RE SICK? YOU LOOK SO WELL (YOU DON'T LOOK SICK)" PERSON

*I'm sorry that I don't look sick enough for you. Would you care to accompany me to the bathroom?* Try to take this as a compliment. Think of it this way: other people look like crap without the excuse of being ill, so well done you.

### THE "I KNOW EXACTLY HOW YOU FEEL/WHAT YOU'RE GOING THROUGH" PERSON

*Do you? Do you have ulcerative colitis? Do you go to the bathroom more than 20 times a day? No? Then you don't have a bloody clue. You really don't. Having diarrhea for one day back in 1997 does not give you even an inkling of how I feel.*

When people say this, they are usually trying to empathize, but it is a narcissistic, superficial empathy that (rightly or wrongly) is annoying as hell.

## THE "YOU'RE SO THIN! I'M SO JEALOUS" PERSON

*Yes. Malnourishment is the BEST. Believe me, if I could trade my colon for yours, I would. And then I would kick your skinny ass.*

## THE "TRY TO RELAX (DON'T GET SO STRESSED) AND EXERCISE MORE" PERSON

*Just. Don't. Better yet, eat a box of laxatives and then run a marathon. Relaxed?*

## THE "YOU HAVE TO GO TO THE BATHROOM AGAIN???" PERSON

*Yes, I do. Did you miss the part where I explained I have a condition I can't control? Or would you rather I squat right here and make my humiliation complete?*

## THE "HAVE YOU TRIED TAKING ALOE JUICE/VITAMIN E/NOT EATING WHEAT?" OR "MAYBE IT'S YOUR DIET" PERSON

*If only the medical community had thought of that first. Here's me having my colon removed like a mug. Please explain to me, in detail, exactly how this works, because we're gonna win a goddamn Nobel prize.*

## THE "YOUR FACE IS SO PUFFY! YOU SHOULD GET MORE SLEEP" PERSON

*My face is puffy because I'm taking large amounts of steroids to try to keep my own immune system from killing me. Also, I was up all night pondering how incredibly rude some people are.*

## THE "SHOULD YOU BE EATING THAT?" PERSON

*Eating what? Food? Which has nothing at all to do with my actual illness? Here, on second thought, you have it. Maybe with your mouth full, you won't be able to be such a busybody.*

## THE "WHY ARE YOU SO TIRED?" PERSON

*I am tired because people keep asking me stupid questions.*

## THE "DO YOU HAVE TO WEAR DIAPERS?" PERSON

*Seriously? Is that any of your business? How often do you masturbate? What? That's too personal?* Although, sometimes this person is genuinely asking out of sympathy. Use your discretion.

## THE "UGH, TOO MUCH DETAIL" PERSON

*You ASKED. If you are nosy enough to want details, then you'd better belt up and ride it out. You've already made me self-conscious by asking me to explain stuff to you in the first place. Don't you dare make me feel awkward for doing so.*

## THE "YOU'RE CANCELING AGAIN?" PERSON

*Yes, I am. I don't want to, but all I'm capable of doing at the moment is sitting here trying to keep warm and not cry myself to sleep. But at least I've now got guilt to keep me company.*

## THE "SO-AND-SO CURED THEIR ULCERATIVE COLITIS BY..." PERSON

*Good for them. Since they didn't have their colon removed, it probably helped that they didn't have ulcerative colitis in the first place.*

## THE "OH MY GOD, CAN YOU HEAR THAT PERSON GOING TO THE BATHROOM? HAHAHA" PERSON

*Yes, I know I sound like a car without a muffler. Uncontrollable diarrhea is hilarious, so thank you for making sure everyone in the vicinity gets to enjoy it. Now run, because that stall door will be opening in 3...2...1 ...*

## THE "AREN'T YOU MAKING A BIG DEAL OVER SOME DIARRHEA?" PERSON

*Are you telling me that if you were going to the toilet up to 40 times per day for weeks at a time, you <u>wouldn't</u> be making a big deal out of it?*

## THE "TUT, TUT, YOU'RE USING THE DISABLED BATHROOM?" PERSON

*Yes, I am. And I am not the least bit ashamed about it. Let me tell you a story...*

## THE "WOW, HAVING ULCERATIVE COLITIS MUST BE THE SHITS LOLOLOLOL" PERSON

*Yes, you can make a lot of puns about poo. It might only be funny the first time you say it, but don't let that stop you. I'm sure the 50th time will be hilarious.*

And the winner:

## THE "ARE YOU SURE YOU'RE NOT JUST HAVING YOUR PERIOD?" PERSON

*I've had my period every month for 18 years. I'm fairly certain that by this point, I can tell the difference between my rectum and my vagina.*

You have been warned.

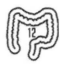

# BITE YOUR LIP AND FAKE IT
## SOCIAL MEDIA

## SOCIAL MEDIA DOS AND DON'TS

Thanks to social media, you can now tell people how you're feeling the minute you feel it; but just because you can, doesn't mean you should. Posting about your illness when you have a chronic condition like ulcerative colitis can be tricky, especially if you have a tendency to post mainly negative comments. Occasionally telling everyone how awful you feel can be comforting—both to vent and get some well-deserved love thrown back your way—but constant status reports on just how hard you have it does both yourself and your friends a disservice. Social media was not created with the sole purpose of providing you with a captive audience for a blow-by-blow account of the trials of your life.

Consider how you view posts on social media. Do you have a friend whose feed consists in large part of complaining about how crappy their life is? Even if their bitching is perfectly justified, after the first few posts and your sympathetic responses, chances are you have begun to dread seeing their name appear on your feed. You may feel resentful at the constant and obvious expectation for you to respond to what seems less like a sharing of feelings and more like an invitation to a self-indulgent pity-party. Since nothing you say seems to make a difference anyway, the whole exercise becomes tiresome, and you struggle to sympathize. Be honest. If you're not already ignoring that person's posts, you're probably considering it. If you don't feel this way, then you're either a saint or lying. And who could blame you? You have your own crap to worry about.

Whether this reaction to another person's hardships is right or wrong is not the point; it's simply how the majority of people feel. While people are happy to extend kindness and compassion to someone they like or love, they also have an understandable desire to carry their own burdens. I'm not saying you shouldn't discuss your illness on social media—you should—but talk about it in a way that is inclusive rather than alienating, and you'll find that people are more than happy to give you the support you need.

## DOS

### BE POSITIVE
Although it can be difficult at times, try to post comments about your illness only if they are positive. Positive posts can include personal milestones you've reached, good news you've received, or goals you've achieved in spite of your illness.

### BE EDUCATIONAL
Bring awareness to your illness as a whole (rather than just your personal experience of it) by posting relevant articles about topics such as new breakthroughs in treatments. People who are genuinely curious will have a look, and those who aren't can bypass them.

### BE FUNNY
Humor is often the best way to let people know how you are feeling without seeming as though you want pity. People enjoy laughing, and having ulcerative colitis is a goldmine for universally-enjoyed potty humor. That said, keep it clever and classy, otherwise people just think you're crude.

### BE HONEST
At the end of the day, be honest with yourself. You're posting about your illness because you want attention and sympathy. That is not a bad thing—you deserve it. But do it sparingly and in a way in which people feel they can be supportive without being obligated to carry you.

## BE PART OF A GROUP

There are social media groups for people with ulcerative colitis. If you need to vent, vent to people who can properly empathize. You may not be special, but you'll be understood.

## BE REALISTIC

Don't post with the sole intention of seeing how many of your friends respond and then measuring your worth against these responses, or lack thereof. Social media is used by people to socialize with minimal effort on their part. Understand it as such.

# DON'TS

## BE SELF-PITYING

Nothing scatters people to the wind like self-pity. Self-deprecation is fine, but self-pity makes people very uncomfortable. You'll get supportive comments back from some people, but many will eventually steer clear of you. Fair? Maybe not, but it's reality.

## BE ANGRY

Like self-pity, anger about your condition makes people very uncomfortable. It's no one's fault that you're ill, not even your own. The universe doesn't give a shit, so there's no point ranting about it.

## BE SELF-ABSORBED

Even if you're posting positive comments about your illness, do so judiciously. People get bored of seeing that crap constantly infiltrating their timelines. You're ill. We get it!

## POST SELF-INDULGENT HOSPITAL SELFIES

Thumbs up after a successful surgery? Good. Pouty face in hospital bed that screams "I need even MORE attention than 24-hour medical care can provide"? Bad.

## TRY TO BAIT SYMPATHY

Read your post aloud before you send it. It can be painfully obvious that you're fishing for attention when you think you're being easy-breezy.

## TAKE IT PERSONALLY

People have their own lives to live and are usually more concerned with that than how many bowel movements you've had today. It's not that they don't care, it's . . . Well, it's that they don't care. It's not personal; it's cat videos.

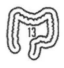

# THE DRUGS DON'T WORK

## A GUIDE TO BEING IN THE HOSPITAL

If your ulcerative colitis is out of control, you'll inevitably end up in the hospital. It doesn't have to be a completely terrible experience, and being prepared will help make your stay a more positive experience for everyone involved.

## HOSPITAL SURVIVAL KIT

### YOUR OWN PAJAMAS
Having your own PJs makes a difference physically and psychologically. It's far more pleasant to lie there in something soft and beautiful that you've picked, rather than an over-starched burlap bag that a hundred people have worn. If morphine makes you adventurous, definitely opt for pajama pants to guarantee your ass is covered.

### WIPES
Although hospitals do have toilet paper, it ain't the good stuff. Plus, you can use the wipes for your hands, your face, etc. if you won't be getting out of bed for a while.

### YOUR OWN COFFEE CUP
Make yourself at home.

## PEN AND PAPER

Just think about how many classics have been written while the authors have been off their tits in a drug-fueled haze. See this as your opportunity.

## COMPUTER

Load it up with movies, TV, games, whatever. Try to make everything available offline, because hospital internet is expensive. If you can then get your eyes to focus, you're golden. If you really want to be online, but don't want to pay, bring mobile WiFi.

## BOOKS, MAGAZINES ETC.

Magazines are especially good since there is usually a roaring trade of swapsies. Don't bring anything too intellectual, however; due to the morphine, chances are you won't remember anything you've read.

## SLIPPERS

Most hospitals are pretty clean. But still. Slippers can be especially useful in a surgical or GI ward—there is sometimes blood and other accidents. Get some with good grips.

## MIRROR, TWEEZERS, MANICURE SET

Being in the hospital may be the only time you get to pamper yourself, so take advantage.

## HAIRBRUSH AND HAIR ACCESSORIES

It's purely psychological. Plus, single doctors and nurses.

## SOAP, SHAMPOO, AND YOUR OWN TOWEL

You can get this stuff from the hospital, but your own is so much better.

## BATHROBE AND SHOWER SHOES

Trying to get dressed again in a wet shower room is the *worst*.

## MENSTRUAL PADS

Yes, the hospital does supply menstrual pads, but unless you enjoy wedging a comically large brick of cotton between your legs, bring your own.

## YOUR TEDDY
Just make sure you wash it when you get home.

## PHOTOS
Photos of your family serve as a memento of what you have to look forward to when you get out. This reminder can help make your hospital stay more bearable, especially if you can't stand some of them.

## A HOBBY OF SOME KIND
You never know how long you may be in the hospital. I became a cross-stitch adept due to the amount of time I spent inside.

## MOISTURIZER
For some reason, hospitals are really damn dry.

## MONEY
For bribes and the mobile snack cart that delivers bedside.

# RULES OF HOSPITAL ETIQUETTE

## YOU ARE NOT STAYING AT A HOTEL
Before you complain about the food, the 'service,' or even the lighting, stop and think about where you are. If you're well enough to complain about everything, you're well enough to go home.

## NURSES ARE NOT SERVANTS
I understand that the uniforms are confusing. I know that you're scared, and you're sick, and you're in pain. So am I. And yet, I don't feel that it gives me the right to be an asshole. If you can haul your ass out of bed and down the hall to have a cigarette, don't soil the bed because it is "the nurse's job" to wipe your ass. Have some respect.

## SHUT UP
I'm avoiding eye contact with you for a reason. The curtain is drawn around my bed for a reason. I'm pretending I'm dead *for a reason.* That reason is that I don't want to talk to you. If you just wanted to say "Hi," great. "Hello!" But you don't. You want to tell me your life story, and you want to hear mine, and I am sorry, but I am just not interested. My sympathy well has run dry. I am tired, and in pain, and I just want to watch *Game of Thrones.*

## HAVING SEX IS NOT APPROPRIATE
Ever.

## TAKE YOUR MEDICATION
Nobody is going to give you a gold star for being tough and not taking your pain meds, but I *will* punch you in the teeth when you start whining because you're what? In pain? Also, NOBODY LIKES HEPARIN. But you'll like a thrombosis even less, I promise.

## DON'T BE MELODRAMATIC
People may die right in front of you. It's sad, and scary, and awful. Don't make it about you and your feelings, *especially* when their loved ones are there.

## WASH

If you can't make it to the shower on your own, get the nurses to help you. I understand that we're all a bit stinky on the GI and surgery wards, but there's a limit. I inadvertently laid in my own filth for two days while temporarily paralyzed after my first surgery, and neither the nurses nor I noticed the smell because the woman in the bed next to mine had refused to wash for *days*.

## YOU'RE NOT THE ONLY PATIENT ON THE WARD

You may be on a ward with patients whose illness is more serious than yours. (Hard to imagine, I know). Make your needs clear, but not every five minutes. The nurses will get to you as soon as they can, if for no better reason than to shut you the hell up.

## DO NOT MAKE YOURSELF UP AND SPEND YOUR TIME TAKING POUTY SELFIES

This makes you look like an asshole at any time, but *especially* at this time.

## A "THANK-YOU" BASKET FOR THE NURSES AFTER YOUR STAY WOULDN'T GO AMISS

And not a crappy fruit basket either.

# HOW TO ENJOY YOUR STAY

## TRY TO THINK OF IT AS A HOLIDAY
You are encouraged to take free narcotics, you get to choose your meals from a menu and have them delivered to your bedside, your linen is changed daily, and you can sleep whenever you want. It may not be the best holiday you've ever had, but you did pay for it in blood, tears, and taxes, right? You might as well enjoy it.

## UNDERSTAND THE SYSTEM
Stock up on breakfast items. Breakfast tends to be the best meal of the day. After that, things can get weird. Fill the drawer in your little nightstand with as many peanut butter packets and bananas as you can, even if you hate bananas.

## BEHOLD THE MYSTERIOUS TAPESTRY OF HUMAN LIFE
Some of the strangest shit you will ever experience will be in the hospital. Roll with it. If a lady thinks you're her husband and tries to get into bed with you, choose to think it's because her husband has fabulous, perky breasts and not because you have a steroid beard. Don't take it personally if she later tries to stab you with a butter knife.

## IT'S HOBBY TIME!
You finally have some free time to enjoy your hobbies. Knit, make lists, or finish Skyrim.

## BINGE WATCH/READ
Catch up on every book, TV show, or movie you always wanted to enjoy.

## WRITE LETTERS
Having to look your mortality in the face may make you re-evaluate your life. Write letters to people and tell them the things you've always wanted to tell them. Especially if you want to tell them you think they're an asshole. They need to know, and you may not get another chance.

## YOU HAVE NO CHORES
Except eat, maybe walk a few steps, and keep yourself clean. Easy.

## YOU HAVE AN ADJUSTABLE BED
Up, down, slanty, flat—lots of people would kill to have one of these at home.

## YOU'LL GET SYMPATHY GIFTS
Everyone who visits you in the hospital feels they should bring gifts, unless they're horrible. Yes, you will probably get a lot of grapes, but you'll get some good stuff too, I promise.

## PRACTICE PASSIVE-AGGRESSION
If you're not fond of the person who is visiting, you can always pretend to fall asleep. Stare into space for a few seconds, mumble, "Thank you so much for coming to see me . . . " and down you go.

## CLOSE YOUR CURTAIN
Enjoy the peace and quiet.

## BOND WITH YOUR FAMILY MEMBERS
Get your significant other to become your shower boy/girl. They'll get to feel helpful, and you'll get to be scrubbed down by someone who has already seen you naked. Try not to look too sexy (see Rules of Hospital Etiquette).

## MAKE FRIENDS, OR NOT
You can meet some very nice, interesting people in the hospital, especially if you share a condition. At the same time, don't feel that you have to be social with anyone. Just focus on getting
yourself ready for the rest of your life.

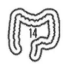

# EYE OF THE TIGER

## TOUGH LOVE RULES FOR SURVIVING ULCERATIVE COLITIS

### YES, YOU HAVE A CHRONIC ILLNESS
Yes, it's awful. Deal with it

### IT'S OKAY TO FEEL SORRY FOR YOURSELF, BUT DON'T BE OBNOXIOUS ABOUT IT
Self-pity is destructive and even worse, boring.

### SYMPATHY IS FICKLE
Don't milk it.

### USE A COMBINATION OF COPING STRATEGIES
Do what works for you, not what other people tell you that you should be doing.

### ACCEPT THAT THERE IS NO IMMEDIATE FIX
Living with ulcerative colitis is an ongoing process, and you will have setbacks, usually when you least expect them.

### TAKE EVERY DAY AS IT COMES
But make plans and set goals for the future.

### YOU ARE NOT SPECIAL
Meaning, you are not alone. There are a lot of us out there.

## DON'T DEFINE YOURSELF BY YOUR DISEASE
Everyone goes through something, even if it's only that their diamond shoes are too tight. The struggle is real.

## BE PROACTIVE
Not being proactive about coping with your condition is a choice that will leave you miserable and isolated, with no one to blame but yourself. Take responsibility for the things you can change.

## PIMP YOUR BATHROOM
You're going to be spending a lot of time in there, so you might as well make it pleasant.

## TAKE YOUR MEDS
There are no gold stars for being a hero; only pain and diarrhea.

## DIAPERS HAVE COME A LONG WAY SINCE YOU FIRST WORE THEM
Use them. Get over it.

## ACCEPT HELP WHEN IT IS OFFERED, BUT HELP YOURSELF WHENEVER YOU CAN
Otherwise, you'll lose your edge, and when the zombie apocalypse happens, you'll be in deep shit of the survivin' kind.

## DON'T TALK ABOUT YOUR ILLNESS ALL OF THE TIME
It's boring.

## BE SELFISH WHEN YOU NEED TO BE
This does not mean all the time.

## YOU ARE MUCH MORE BOTHERED ABOUT THE WAY YOUR BODY LOOKS/SOUNDS/SMELLS THAN ANYONE ELSE
Really.

**FORCE YOURSELF TO GO OUT**

You will probably have fun. Also, if you don't, people will eventually stop asking.

**REMEMBER:**

If you're not feeling even a tiny bit of illness, pain, nausea, sadness, anger, fatigue, irritation, or itchiness ...

# IT'S BECAUSE YOU'RE DEAD.

# ACKNOWLEDGEMENTS

Big love to my family for their support: Jamie, my Mr. Darcy (only, without the grand estate, fine manners, and riding breeches). Thank you for never letting me feel sorry for myself. I love you. Harlan, who is the symbol of our victory. Peter and Kal, for being both our family and best friends, and for laughing at me in the right way. My dads, Ralph and Alan, who take everything in their stride and always offer to buy the first round. My mother Lynne, who traveled thousands of miles to become my caregiver decades after she had thought she was done. My other mother Val, who shared a seat on this bus to hell. Colin and Denny, whose friendship and courage tempered my heart. And to Emily, my parabatai: we both look good in black. I could have written this book without all of you, but it probably would have been terrible.

Thank you to everyone who has battled ulcerative colitis and didn't suffer in silence. Your failure, your success, and your humor inspired me.

Extra thanks to Peter Cross for his endless patience and skill in creating everything I need, and to Mia Darien, for her quick and thorough eye.

And finally, a slow clap for my medical team: some of you were amazing; some of you were infuriating. Either way, we got there in the end.

# APPENDIX

## SURVIVAL KIT CHECKLISTS

*For printable checklists, go to screamingmeemie.com

### FISTULA SURVIVAL KIT CHECKLIST

- ☐ wet wipes
- ☐ barrier cream
- ☐ absorption pad
- ☐ change of underwear
- ☐ disposal bags
- ☐ hand sanitizer
- ☐ change of dressing
- ☐ mirror
- ☐ scissors
- ☐ cushion
- ☐ odor-neutralizing spray

# ULCERATIVE COLITIS SURVIVAL KIT CHECKLIST

- ☐ wipes
- ☐ vaseline®
- ☐ mentholated lotion
- ☐ antidiarrheals
- ☐ painkillers
- ☐ change of clothes
- ☐ change
- ☐ scent spray
- ☐ books and magazines
- ☐ pantyliners
- ☐ tissues
- ☐ snacks
- ☐ drinks
- ☐ pictures of your loved ones
- ☐ antibacterial hand wipes/gel
- ☐ notepad & paper
- ☐ moisturizer
- ☐ trick shoes
- ☐ a list including your condition, medications, and doctor's details

# HOSPITAL SURVIVAL KIT CHECKLIST

- ☐ pajamas
- ☐ wipes
- ☐ coffee cup
- ☐ pen and paper
- ☐ computer
- ☐ books, magazines, etc.
- ☐ slippers
- ☐ mirror, tweezers, manicure set
- ☐ hairbrush and accessories
- ☐ soap
- ☐ shampoo
- ☐ towel
- ☐ bathrobe
- ☐ shower shoes
- ☐ menstrual pads
- ☐ teddy
- ☐ photos
- ☐ hobby supplies
- ☐ moisturizer
- ☐ money

# GLOSSARY

**aminosalicylates:** Also known as 5-ASAs, these medications are prescribed to help reduce inflammation in your colon. Common examples include **sulfasalazine** (Azulfidine®, Salazopyrin®, Sulazine®), **mesalamine** (Asacol®, Canasa®, Lialda®, Mezavant®, Pentasa®, Rowasa®, Salofalk®), **olsalazine** (Dipentum®), and **balsalazide** (Colazal®, Colazide®). Aminosalicylates are available as tablets, suppositories, and enemas.

**antibiotics:** A type of medication prescribed to treat infection. The ones most commonly prescribed in treating ulcerative colitis-related infections include **metronidazole** (Flagyl®), **ciprofloxacin** (Cipro®), **vancomycin** (Vancocin®), and rifaximin (Xifaxan®).

**biologic therapy:** Medication for severe ulcerative colitis that has been genetically engineered to suppresses specific parts of your immune system. **Infliximab** (Remicade®), **adalimumab** (Humira®), and **golimumab** (Simponi®) are examples of biologics.

**colon:** Also known as the large bowel, large intestine, or the devil's playground.

**colonoscopy:** The secret handshake of our exclusive club. A slim, flexible tube is inserted into your rectum and through your large intestine, allowing your gastroenterologist to have a long, hard look.

**corticosteroids:** The class of steroids used to treat ulcerative colitis, and which made Bruce Banner the man he is today.

**diarrhea:** Bowel movements that are loose, watery, unformed. Whatever. Definitely not solid. You will become very familiar with this word, but you'll still have trouble spelling it.

**enema:** Keep your friends close, but your enemas closer. Awkward, but worth it. Foam or liquid, enemas are inserted into your rectum to deliver medication straight to your colon.

**flare:** Not as fun as it sounds. A flare is when your ulcerative colitis is in full swing. Also called a flare-up.

**gastroenterologist:** A specialist that will diagnose and treat your disease; you'll either love them or hate them.

**immunomodulators:** Medications used to alter the function of your immune system. Usually immunosuppressants, these chemical treatments are intended to limit the ability of your immune system to attack you. Azathioprine (Azasan®, Imuran®), and 6-mercaptopurine (Purinethol®, Purixam®) are the two you may become familiar with.

**inflammation:** The reaction of the body to injury. In ulcerative colitis, inflammation occurs as your T-cells infiltrate and damage your colon, resulting in pain and tissue swelling.

**perianal skin:** The skin around your anus. Potentially a source of great anguish.

**remission:** The state between flares in which your UC is no longer active. Considered by many to be a myth.

**suppository:** A wax rocket that you insert up your butt and make a game of seeing how long you can keep it in. An admittedly efficient way of delivering medication to your rectum.

# INDEX

## M

malnutrition, 10

mouth sores, 10

## N

nausea, 9, 74

## P

pain, 9-10, 73

pelvic floor exercise, 50–51

physical consequences of ulcerative
colitis, **9–17**

pregnancy, **77–79**

after birth, 79

before pregnancy, 77–78

during pregnancy, 78

giving birth, 78

probiotics, **40–41**

## R

RADAR key, 18

relationships and ulcerative colitis, **68–72**

## S

sex and ulcerative colitis, **73–76**

emotional changes and issues, 74

physical changes and issues, 73–74

tips for sex with ulcerative colitis, 74–
76

side effects, 10

social events, **57–58**

social media, **91–94**

survival kits, **21-25, 26-27, 95-97**

fistula, 26–27

hospital survival kit, 95–97

ulcerative colitis, 21–25

## T

the people you'll meet, **87–90**

tough love rules for surviving ulcerative
colitis, **103–5**

travel, **53–56**

before you go, 53–54

in the car, 55–57

on the plane, 54–55

once you're there, 56

## U

ulcerative colitis

access to public bathrooms, **18**

and the people you'll meet, **87–90**

being in the hospital, **95–101**

bulking, **38–39**

cons, 5–6

diet and, **31–36**

emotional impact of, **59–67**

exercise and, **47–51**

fashion and, **81–83**

hair and, **84–86**

healthcare professionals and, **43–46**

physical consequences of, **9–12, 17**

pregnancy and, **77–79**

probiotics, **40–41**

pros, 6–8

relationships and, **68–72**

sex and, **73–76**

social events and, **57–58**

social media and, **91–94**

survival kit, **21–25**

tough love rules for surviving, **103–5**

travel and, **53–56**

# W

weight fluctuations, 10